Food Insecurity on Campus

Food Insecurity on Campus

Action and Intervention

EDITED BY

Katharine M. Broton and Clare L. Cady

Foreword by Sara Goldrick-Rab

JOHNS HOPKINS UNIVERSITY PRESS | *Baltimore*

Johns Hopkins University Press
2715 North Charles Street
Baltimore, Maryland 21218-4363
www.press.jhu.edu

Library of Congress Cataloging-in-Publication Data

Names: Broton, Katharine M., 1983– editor. | Cady, Clare L., 1980– editor.
Title: Food insecurity on campus : action and intervention / edited by
    Katharine M. Broton and Clare L. Cady ; foreword by Sara Goldrick-Rab.
Description: Baltimore : Johns Hopkins University Press, 2020. |
    Includes bibliographical references and index.
Identifiers: LCCN 2019031150 | ISBN 9781421437729 (paperback) |
    ISBN 9781421437736 (ebook)
Subjects: LCSH: Food security—United States. | College students—
    United States—Social conditions.
Classification: LCC HD9005 .F65825 2020 | DDC 363.8/830973—dc23
LC record available at https://lccn.loc.gov/2019031150

A catalog record for this book is available from the British Library.

Special discounts are available for bulk purchases of this book.
For more information, please contact Special Sales at
specialsales@press.jhu.edu.

Johns Hopkins University Press uses environmentally friendly book materials,
including recycled text paper that is composed of at least 30 percent post-
consumer waste, whenever possible.

CONTENTS

Dropping out of college is nothing new. Ever since people began attending college, some students have left without degrees. But the consequences of non-completion have grown more substantial. These days it is hard to have a stable income or access to a decent job without at least some education after high school. College prices have become so substantial, and financial aid so scarce, that loans are often required. Leaving college in debt without a degree is frequently painful, and sometimes financially ruinous.

Higher education is therefore gradually accepting greater responsibility for increasing the rates of college completion. In order to succeed, colleges will need to consider *all* the conditions that facilitate college success. This used to simply mean considering the academic preparation students bring to college, the information they possess about how to navigate school, and their knowledge of financial aid. But times have changed. The new economics of college have greatly increased the gaps between college costs, family resources, and financial aid.[1] Even working students receiving financial aid are falling short of the funds needed to secure their basic needs.

That is what makes this book so important. Food insecurity is now common on American college campuses. Researchers have documented this fact repeatedly over the past decade, and the United States Government Accountability Office recently affirmed it.[2] But what can and should colleges do about it? What can and should policymakers do? Will the initial movement to create campus food pantries evolve to push beyond "sweet charity" and engage more just efforts to empower students and meet their needs in a sustainable way?[3] Will we address the root causes of campus hunger or only treat symptoms of the trauma?

I teach at an urban public university—a Research 1, top of the Carnegie rankings. I'm not one of Philadelphia's schoolteachers; I am a professor with just one class to teach each term and a big research budget. But those trappings of prestige no longer shield me or my colleagues from the realities of poverty in our city, and more importantly they do not help my students. And I am not alone.

Since 2008, my team's studies of how students finance college have revealed that tuition is not the main barrier to degree completion. The first time I met an undergraduate who had not eaten in two days, I was stunned. Now, having conducted numerous studies on the topic and interviewed dozens of homeless college students, I alternate between numb and angry. The best estimates suggest that food insecurity affects as many as one in two college students (three times the rate in the general population); just as many struggle with housing insecurity, and a significant number are homeless. Yet this remains a largely invisible problem, hidden from public view. Stereotypes of ramen noodle diets and couch-surfing partiers prevent us from seeing it. But it is time to get real and admit that we in higher education have a serious problem.

"Any student who has difficulty affording groceries or accessing sufficient food to eat every day or who lacks a safe and stable place to live, and believes this may affect their performance in the course, is urged to contact the Dean of Students for support. Furthermore, please notify me if you are comfortable in doing so. This will enable me to provide any other resources that I may possess."

This is a basic needs security statement that appears on my syllabus, and it represents my challenge to higher education. Can we move beyond grading students and marking down their absences? Can we instead begin to establish a culture of care that will be transmitted and reflected throughout the university?

There are reasons for hope, and many of those reasons are contained in the pages of this book. While they have many limitations, food pantries represent at least an institutional acknowledgment of food insecurity. The College and University Food Bank Alliance (discussed in chap. 2) has more than 700 members from coast to coast, with pantries housed at community colleges and universities, public and private. This is a stunning increase, since in 2012 there were just over 10. Food pantries provide emergency assistance to the students who are lucky enough to know about them, and what they provide varies. Sometimes there are fresh fruits and vegetables, but usually there are cans and bags, some bread, and once in a while there are toiletries too.

Some colleges are moving beyond food pantries. Just over two dozen schools operate a program known as Swipe Out Hunger (described in chap. 5), which reallocates unused dollars on meal plans to students who need them. Single Stop and other homegrown efforts are helping students apply for the Supplemental Nutrition Assistance Program (SNAP; discussed in chap. 6), and some institutions are beginning to accept Electronic Benefit Transfer (EBT) on campus. In Houston, the local food bank is offering "food scholarships" to community college students, proactively providing groceries rather than waiting for emergencies to occur. There are food recovery networks, nutrition programs, and educational activities like Challah for Hunger (highlighted in chap. 4), where students gather to break bread, learn about poverty, and engage in actions to address it on campuses. These efforts are entry points to systemic change and make it possible to envision a time in which the National School Lunch Program will operate on all campuses, providing breakfast and lunch to every student who needs it.

We have to push further, however, if we want to end campus hunger and help students complete degrees. It is very difficult to learn anything—whether in a vocational training program for a welding certificate, working toward an associate degree in nursing, or in a philosophy class—without first having your basic needs met. Many inefficiencies of the current higher education system are discussed throughout Washington, DC, and the nation, but no actions are taken to address them. Instead, they are ignored while students struggle. The authors of this book know that college is an exceptional route out of poverty, but for that path to work, students must escape the conditions of poverty long enough to complete their degrees. I am excited about the actions and approaches these contributors describe, and most of all the challenges they ask us to consider. Addressing campus hunger has the potential to help individual students, but it also contains the possibility of doing more— of transforming higher education into a more effective environment that facilitates greater learning. Please use this volume as you engage in that work.

Sara Goldrick-Rab
Founding Director,
Hope Center for College, Community, and Justice
Professor of Higher Education Policy and Sociology,
Temple University

Notes

1. Sara Goldrick-Rab, *Paying the Price: College Costs, Financial Aid, and the Betrayal of the American Dream* (Chicago: University of Chicago Press, 2016).

2. United States Government Accountability Office, *Food Insecurity: Better Information Could Help Eligible College Students Access Federal Food Assistance Benefits*, GAO-19-95 (Washington, DC: Author, Published Dec. 2018 and Publicly Released Jan. 2019), https://www.gao.gov/products /GAO-19-95.

3. Janet Poppendieck, *Sweet Charity? Emergency Food and the End of Entitlement* (London: Penguin Books, 1999).

This book represents the talents and energies of many practitioners and scholars who have shaped the field of basic needs insecurities through research, practice, and policy. As the editors, we wish to offer thanks to those without whom this book would not be possible—the people and institutions seeking to ensure that all students can not only access higher education but also thrive in the pursuit of their goals.

To authors of the foreword and book chapters: Dr. Sara Goldrick-Rab, Dr. Michael Rosen, Talia Berday-Sacks, James Dubick, Rachel Sumekh, Sarah Crawford, Nicole Hindes, Dr. Denise Woods-Bevly, Dr. Sabrina Sanders, Dr. Jennifer Maguire, Dr. Rashida Crutchfield, Dr. Russel Lowery-Hart, Cara Crowley, Jordan Herrera, Amy Ellen Duke-Benfield, and Samuel Chu—your time, energy, and expertise are invaluable to our field. You are the leaders of this work, and we are grateful to you for sharing these with us and with our readers. This book would not be possible without you.

To those who advised on content: Ruben Canedo, Dr. Daphne Hernandez, Jessica Bartholow, Nate Smith-Tyge, Brandon Mathews, and Sonal Chauhan Patel—you also are engaging in positive movement toward the goal of alleviating student food insecurity. Thank you for your thoughts and contributions, which ensure that this book is accurate and provides the best information possible to readers.

To our home institutions: the University of Iowa College of Education and the College and University Food Bank Alliance—you provide us with a powerful place and platform to engage in this work. Thank you for your support of our goal to put this book together.

To our families and partners—you support who we are and the goals we set. Thank you for love and patience as we work through challenges and deadlines to pursue excellence. Our lives are better with you in them, and we are grateful for you.

Finally, to the students whose lives are impacted by food insecurity—thank you for your persistence and your resilience. Please know that we are working as fast as possible to solve this problem, and we acknowledge and honor your struggles and pain. It is our hope that this book serves to improve your lives and the lives of those students coming after you.

Introduction

KATHARINE M. BROTON AND CLARE L. CADY

This book is a direct response to the requests that we, the editors and chapter contributors, have received for guidance and support in addressing hunger and food insecurity on college campuses. Together, we seek to improve efforts to support students and, ultimately, end hunger and food insecurity among college students. We envision this volume as part of an iterative process, drawing on those who came before us while guiding others who come after us. At a time of increasing awareness and interest in addressing the problem of food insecurity in higher education, this book provides the latest and most promising solutions from leaders and innovators in the field. We make no claim to have discovered the issue of food insecurity on college campuses, nor do we believe that this issue is new. However, we are actively involved in the growing number of studies and interventions focused on understanding it as a phenomenon and addressing it as a threat to college success. Our goals are twofold: provide a venue for college, community, and policy leaders to share the lessons they have learned in the fight to end student hunger, and compile a comprehensive source of information, guidance, and support for those seeking to develop an intervention or strategy. It is our hope that by publishing this book we can decrease the time from "interest" to "action" and better serve more students more quickly.

Multiple Approaches to Supporting Students

Beyond making it simpler to identify and develop a single intervention, this volume demonstrates the importance of addressing campus food insecurity in a coordinated and strategic manner. There is no one perfect intervention, no silver bullet, that when initiated will end student hunger on a single campus, let alone multiple campuses. Each action or intervention has benefits as well as limitations and must be shaped to fit a particular context. Among programmatic interventions, for example, food pantries are critical to addressing student hunger today. Their strength lies in the ability to respond quickly and reactively in emergency situations. Yet they only provide a small amount of food at a discrete point in time, serving more as a bandage to address acute need rather than a long-term, sustaining solution. A different programmatic approach is to help connect eligible students with existing public benefits such as the Supplemental Nutrition Assistance Program (SNAP, formerly known as food stamps), which provides them with funds they can use to purchase food each month. While these additional resources can prevent students from becoming food insecure, this intervention also has limitations. It takes time and energy to navigate the complex enrollment process; students may have to wait weeks to get their first Electronic Benefit Transfer (EBT) disbursements, and they may not be able to use their EBT card on campus. This program is also contingent on political support, leaving its existence and availability vulnerable to change. Given that each intervention or action has distinct pros and cons, we encourage campuses to consider a more holistic approach, rather than focus on a single intervention. A holistic approach stitches together a suite of strategies tailored to a particular community. Given the diversity of food insecurity experiences on college campuses nationwide, the intervention strategies described in this volume may be more effective in combination with one another and existing local efforts.

We see the value in how specific communities—including students, faculty, staff, administrators, faith leaders, and charitable organizations—can be leveraged and coordinated to address student hunger. Student activism is a powerful catalyst for social change and can be the tipping point for campus action, but the movement it generates can wane when student leaders graduate or move on to other projects. Faculty can band together, bringing their expertise, regular contact with students, and ability to organize (especially if unionized) in order to gather resources to help students. Administrators can provide visionary leadership and develop a culture of caring for students. This work is not easy, however, and there are always competing demands for time and resources. We believe that breaking down silos and harnessing the power of these groups in an integrated and institutionalized manner has the most potential to create lasting change for students. Though this volume focuses on a selection of the most promising actions and interventions, we take a broad and inclusive view of the communities and strategies that can help end hunger on college campuses.

We also challenge our readers to think beyond programs and also consider how research and policy can be combined and coordinated with practice to promote food security. For instance, research can describe the scope of the problem and implications for student success, provide legitimacy, and serve as an initial strategy that spurs direct programmatic or policy actions. Policy change and culture change are critical to addressing the roots of student hunger, stopping the problem before it starts. These actions have their own limitations as well, including that they can take a long time to reach students. We recommend that these actions be used in concert with programs to address student hunger in the present and prevent it in the future.

Choosing the "Right" Actions and Interventions

This volume has a diverse set of contributing authors who are working to address food insecurity in higher education from different vantage points. The editorial partnership of an academic researcher and an experienced practitioner serves as the first step to ensuring representation of multiple perspectives. Dr. Katharine Broton is a sociologist of education and one of the first scholars to study food insecurity and hunger on college campuses. In her research, she uses multiple methods to examine the role of poverty and inequality in higher education, as well as policies and programs designed to minimize related disparities and promote college and socioeconomic success. Clare Cady has spent the better part of the past decade designing and implementing food insecurity interventions, including campus pantries, food vouchers and stipends, SNAP enrollment programs, and partnerships with campus dining centers. In 2012, she took the work to scale, cofounding the College and University Food Bank Alliance with her colleague Nate Smith-Tyge from Michigan State University.

We believe that research is enhanced when it is informed by those whom it affects and that, conversely, practice and policy are improved when informed by research. Together, the iterative combination of research, practice, and policy is one of the best ways to effect positive change. It is in this spirit that we draw on our unique strengths and perspectives to bring together a collection of chapters that provide a snapshot of the current movement to end college student hunger in the United States. To be clear, we (the editors) do not necessarily agree with all of the arguments made by each contributing author—and we doubt they would all agree with one another—but we respect their work and believe that the inclusion of their voice positively contributes to the pursuit of our common goal. When determining which strategies to include in this volume, we considered the following four aspects.

Target Focus

We only include strategies that can directly impact food insecurity among college students. We include interventions where the sole program focus is on food security, such as on-campus food pantries and meal swipe donation programs, as well as interventions that take a broader approach to fighting basic needs insecurity, including emergency aid programs and wraparound services that provide a range of supports related to food, housing, transportation, childcare, and other needs. We include those in the latter category because experiences of food insecurity rarely occur in isolation; students struggling with hunger are often struggling to secure other basic needs. Indeed, many of the chapter authors discuss food and housing insecurity in tandem given the interrelated and interconnected aspects of poverty.[1]

Replication

We only include strategies that have been implemented in multiple higher education contexts. In some cases, a single intervention has been intentionally replicated on multiple campuses as a system or organization scaled their approach. In other cases, similar approaches independently emerged at different institutions or were replicated independently as institutions shared and learned from one another. We believe that strategies implemented similarly but in different contexts may provide the most promising approaches to fighting hunger on college campuses.[2]

Data Driven

We only include programs that demonstrate a commitment to using data and research in their initial design and further development and improvement. The programs we selected for this volume do at least one of the following: cite and utilize existing data on student food insecurity to justify their approach, generate data as they implement their intervention to evaluate and improve their work, and/or adjust how they approach their work in response to new data and evidence in the field.

Variation

Finally, we include approaches that operate across implementation level (federal, state, and local), institutional sector (two- and four-year, public and private), and geographic location. We also chose approaches designed and implemented by people of various backgrounds with different perspectives and professional training. Rather than present a single coordinated strategy, we provide a collection of promising approaches. Food insecurity is a multifaceted problem that requires a multipronged solution. There is a role for each one of us to play, but it is up to you, the reader, to shape and apply these ideas to your particular setting and context.

Limitations of This Book

As we consider the contributions and drawbacks of each action or intervention, we would be remiss in not doing the same for this book. First, the issue of student hunger is not new, and programs to alleviate it predate the current movement to address food insecurity on college campuses.[3] This book does not capture the full history of the work and does not include all of the approaches or ideas within the movement. Our goal is to address a growing and increasingly urgent call for information on how to end student hunger, using common questions and approaches as the core of the information provided. This is the first book dedicated to compiling, organizing, and describing key strategies currently being implemented in the field.

Second, the efficacy of the strategies in this book has not been rigorously evaluated. This is not because we do not value research but because, at the time of writing, rigorous studies of higher education food insecurity interventions do not yet exist.[4] As the movement to end student hunger has grown and strategies to address it have diversified, efforts to evaluate the efficacy of these interventions and their impacts on student success and development have not kept pace. Most evaluation efforts consist of short student feedback forms or testimonials asserting the perceived impact of a particular program. This type of information is often crucial to program development and service improvement. However, it does little to help us understand the trade-offs or cost-effectiveness of different approaches, or which interventions work best for which types of students in which contexts. Currently, there is a growing body of research and evaluation efforts designed to answer such questions. At the time of writing this book, there are two randomized control trials, long considered the gold standard in research, in the field designed to evaluate the causal impacts of food scholarships and meal vouchers on student success and well-being.[5]

Though the field currently lacks rigorous evidence on *what works*, it is clear that hunger is associated with poorer academic and student development outcomes.[6] This intuitive understanding, combined with exposure to student reports of food insecurity, has led higher educational professionals, students, and community partners to take action and respond to students in need today. All of the contributors to this book know students who would not have been able to persist or graduate had they not gotten some form of assistance. It is because of this sense of urgency that we chose to provide guidance that precedes rigorous causal evidence. The need is great, and colleges and universities will continue to implement food security programs—even as we evaluate the work—so we are choosing to provide institutions with information designed to help them implement and refine strategies already in place in the field. It is our position that it is more ethical and productive to share the promising practices and lessons learned that we currently possess to help shape the movement rather than wait for research to catch up.

Overview of the Book

We have organized the chapters to build on one another, describing more discrete interventions earlier in the volume and broader, more comprehensive actions in later chapters. Programs like campus pantries and emergency aid interventions may be the reason one picks up this book, and leading with these strategies will help draw readers toward a broader and more nuanced understanding of student food insecurity as they progress through the volume. We also recognize that this volume may be used in part for courses, for professional development opportunities, or as a guide for new programs. It is for this reason that we, as editors, have included a brief prologue for each chapter that contextualizes its importance within the field of practice.

The first two chapters provide a frame for this book, offering insights from current research and popular practice. First, coeditor Dr. Katharine Broton provides an overview of food insecurity on college campuses, highlighting the relationship between food insecurity and student success. This chapter provides foundational information on the topic, offering readers the opportunity to understand the issue through the latest research. Coeditor Clare Cady builds on this in chapter 2 by describing the phenomenon of campus pantries at colleges as a popular intervention and a gateway to more comprehensive approaches to addressing food insecurity among students. These chapters connect research and practice to provide a wide-ranging perspective on the movement and its history.

Chapters 3-6 include initiatives driven by specific stakeholders: faculty, students, administrators, and nonprofit organizations. In chapter 3, Dr. Michael Rosen shares a faculty-led approach to student poverty and economic crisis; the Faculty and Students Together (FAST) Fund is an emergency aid program that affects students' food security by meeting needs not currently covered by higher education or social services. This chapter also demonstrates the power of faculty unions in addressing student needs. Chapter 4 highlights the potential of student activism in addressing hunger on campuses. James Dubick and Talia Berday-Sacks discuss the history of student movements, providing deeper insights into the work of Challah for Hunger and the National Student Campaign Against

Hunger and Homelessness. In chapter 5, Rachel Sumekh of Swipe Out Hunger provides a case study of a powerful student-led approach. Her personal account of growing Swipe Out Hunger from a group of students donating food from their dining center to a national nonprofit organization also illustrates the critical importance of students and administrators partnering to create change. This is followed by chapter 6, in which Sarah Crawford and Nicole Hindes discuss the ways colleges and universities can create social service programs that integrate on- and off-campus resources to take a holistic and targeted approach to addressing students' basic needs. They highlight two distinct ways to do this: one a homegrown program, the Human Services Resource Center at Oregon State University, and one a national nonprofit, Single Stop. Both programs utilize wraparound services to address student needs, harnessing local, state, and federal resources through intentional networks of partnerships with campus offices, nonprofit organizations, and government agencies.

Chapters 7 and 8 serve as a case study for how an entire system of colleges can take collective action to address food insecurity among their students. In chapter 7, Drs. Denise Woods-Bevly and Sabrina Sanders from the California State University (CSU) Office of the Chancellor discuss how the CSU leveraged data to allocate resources and take action to address food insecurity across all 23 campuses. This chapter underscores the importance of leadership and intentional planning in meeting students' basic needs and fighting food insecurity. This is paired with chapter 8, in which their faculty colleagues, Drs. Jennifer Maguire and Rashida Crutchfield, discuss how research and the data it generates not only are informative but also can serve as foundational drivers for action and change. They explain the ways in which this has occurred across the CSU, with faculty playing a critical role in building the case for the practical action described by Drs. Woods-Bevly and Sanders.

Chapters 9 and 10 focus on broad approaches to student food insecurity that go beyond the campus and its partnerships. Chapter 9 highlights the No Excuses Poverty Initiative at Amarillo College, in which Dr. Russel Lowery-Hart, Cara Crowley, and Jordan Herrera discuss the importance of the community college not only as a catalyst for campus change but also as a hub for the region and its growth. They describe the history of their initiative, including the strategic redesign of campus infrastructure and culture that they undertook to focus on the needs of students as part of a broader community initiative. And finally, in chapter 10 Amy Ellen Duke-Benfield and Samuel Chu provide insights into how policy change can impact student food insecurity by seeking to proactively address its root causes and create overarching solutions. They provide information on national policy approaches and an in-depth look at the ways in which the state of California is leveraging policy to address the needs of students.

To conclude, we, the coeditors, discuss the future of the work, sharing information on emerging initiatives and approaches not addressed in earlier chapters. We provide insights into where the field should be going, including the critical importance of forgoing siloed or boutique programs for coordinated systemic approaches. We also reflect on what is needed to reach these goals at multiple levels, including calls for new research, resources, and actions that will push us forward in the fight to end hunger and food insecurity on our nation's college campuses.

Notes

1. Though federal financial aid is intended to cover students' room and board, we exclude this intervention in this volume since it is widely discussed in other books and articles.

2. Here the term *replication* includes duplication of a broad strategy (e.g., food pantry, emergency grant aid, meal voucher) in addition to the exact reproduction of a particular program or intervention.

3. A recent survey from the College and University Food Bank Alliance found colleges reporting having food pantries on campus to serve students as early as the 1980s. See Sara Goldrick-Rab, Clare Cady, and Vanessa Coca, *Campus Food Pantries: Insights from a National Survey* (Philadelphia: Hope Center for College, Community, and Justice, 2018), https://hope4college .com/wp-content/uploads/2018/10/2018-CUFBA-Report-web3.pdf.

4. Note that there are rigorous intervention studies in other contexts, including K–12 education and the general public, that provide the foundation for many of the interventions used in the higher education context.

5. For more information on these studies, see Sara Goldrick-Rab, Katharine Broton, and Daphne Hernandez, *Addressing Basic Needs Security in Higher Education: An Introduction to Three Evaluations of Supports for Food and Housing at Community Colleges* (Madison: Wisconsin HOPE Lab, 2017), https://hope4college.com/wp-content/uploads/2018/09/Addressing-Basic -Needs-Security-in-Higher-Education.pdf.

6. See chap. 1 for more information.

[1]

Food Insecurity in Higher Education

KATHARINE M. BROTON

Editors' Prologue. This chapter provides an introduction to the problem of food insecurity among college students. Challenging outdated and stereotypical notions of undergraduates, it describes the context of today's college environment, including the ways in which students negotiate the rising net price of college attendance. The chapter explains the difference between food insecurity and hunger, the latest research about the scope and depth of food insecurity among undergraduates, and implications for student success and development. It concludes with a discussion of the potential consequences for failing to respond to the threat of basic needs insecurity in higher education.

About the Author. Katharine M. Broton is an assistant professor of higher education in the Department of Educational Policy and Leadership Studies and the Department of Sociology (courtesy) at the University of Iowa. She is a leading scholar of food insecurity in higher education, and her current research program examines the prevalence of basic needs insecurity among college students, how such insecurity is related to college success, and ways to improve students' material well-being and promote college and socioeconomic success. Her work has appeared in *Educational Researcher, Educational Evaluation and Policy Analysis,* and the *New York Times* and on Wisconsin Public Television, among others. Broton earned her PhD in sociology from the University of Wisconsin–Madison, where she worked with the Wisconsin HOPE Lab.

Michelle is a young African American woman who attends one of the largest and most diverse community colleges in Massachusetts.[1] Her love of gaming and an encouraging high school computer teacher inspired her to pursue a career in computer programming. We met in her college's one-stop office, which provides wraparound case management services for students in need. I was there to learn more about the college's meal voucher program for a research study, and Michelle was a participant who had agreed to meet with me.[2] She was sitting in the waiting area, coloring with Annabel, her 4-year-old daughter. When I walked in, she jumped up with a big smile on her face, outstretched her arm, and apologized as we shook hands. She explained that there had been a last-minute change in Annabel's schedule that required her to pick up Annabel during our earlier scheduled appointment time, but she was ready to talk now.

Michelle took Annabel's hand, and the three of us slowly made our way downstairs to an empty office. Brightly colored signs indicated that the college uses the office to provide free tax preparation services for students, but there were no tax accountants on hand that day. After getting Annabel settled with her coloring book and crayons, Michelle told me about her path to college. She gushed about the goals she has for herself and her family, including a dream of putting her design skills to use in the gaming industry. When I asked her how she pays for college, she said that financial aid covers her tuition and fees. "And how are you paying for your food and your housing and your transportation?" I added. Michelle's mood changed as she tensed up, dropped her head slightly, and quietly responded, "Well, those kinds of things—at first I didn't have." She went on to explain how things started to change—for the better— after she visited her college's one-stop office.

They told me how to get my food stamp card. So they told me what to do, and then I went to the office down in Quincy, and then they helped me out, and I got my food stamp card. And it was only for me. I didn't put Annabel *on it. I didn't know I can put her on it. So I was only getting like $125 and I had to feed both me, her, and my girlfriend, so that wasn't enough.*

—Michelle

With $125 in monthly Supplemental Nutrition Assistance Program (SNAP) benefits, Michelle said, "I would only focus on [Annabel] to make sure she ate most. So I'd get a lot of kid things so that she can eat breakfast stuff—so that she'll eat. And I'd have a little piece out of it." Like so many moms, Michelle was cutting and skipping meals so that she could put the basic needs of her child before her own.[3]

Lack of food combined with little sleep, given her overnight work schedule, meant that Michelle was coming to school exhausted each morning. "I was coming here tired; I would drift off sometimes during my math class," she said. Michelle knew that her situation was not sustainable, but she was not ready to give up on her higher education goals, so she went back to her college's one-stop office. She learned that if she added Annabel to her SNAP application, she would be eligible for additional benefits. The college also provided her with a $300 meal card to use in the college cafeteria. The meal card program is part of her college's comprehensive plan to fight hunger and just one of a number of strategic investments, including a food pantry and emergency aid, designed to help students make ends meet.[4]

Michelle told me, "After I got the [college cafeteria] meal card and everything, it's been going smoothly. I've been eating. I've gained some weight too. I just had a [physical fitness] test, and they do height and weight, and I was 121 [pounds], and now I'm 128 [pounds]. So I've gained." At five feet eight inches tall, Michelle is no longer officially underweight,[5] but she still says, "I'm pretty low [weight], but I'm getting up there, I'm getting up there." Michelle now considers herself "stable," thanks to the combination of SNAP benefits and the college cafeteria meal card. Both are necessary because, as she says, "I can't use my SNAP here" at college "and I mostly buy groceries for Annabel, so all the [SNAP] is used up." Looking back at her first year in college, she says that these food supports "really saved me because I was really going underweight." Michelle will almost surely have more obstacles to overcome before she can become a computer programmer, but she attributes food assistance programs to helping her get through her first year of college.

Experiences of Today's College Students

Michelle, like the majority of her peers, constantly juggles multiple work and family obligations while attending college. Nationally, three-quarters of today's undergraduates are "nontraditional" or "new-traditional" students, meaning they do not fit the stereotype of a young adult, attending college full-time immediately after high school.[6] Approximately two-thirds of undergraduates work while enrolled in college, one-quarter are student parents, half are financially independent according to the financial aid system, nearly half attend school part-time, and one-third delayed college enrollment by a year or more.[7] Just 14 percent of students live on campus while enrolled in college.[8] In reality, students' lives are much more complex than idealized notions of college as a protected time for emergent adulthood.

Over the past three decades, the price of college has increased while the purchasing power of financial aid has not kept pace. According to one estimate, the average annual price of college—including tuition and fees, room and board, books and supplies, transportation, and other expenses—for in-district or in-state students is nearly $18,000 at public two-year colleges and more than $25,000 at public four-year colleges and universities.[9] Approximately 40 percent of undergraduates receive a Pell Grant, the nation's flagship need-based financial aid program to help students from low-income families pay for college, but it does not stretch as far as it once did since the price of college has increased faster than the value of the grant.[10] The maximum Pell Grant is worth nearly

$6,000, meaning that it covers only a fraction of the total price of college attendance.[11] Furthermore, the financial aid system fails to accurately reflect the daily realities of today's students. Recent research indicates that the financial needs analysis systematically overstates the amount of money students are able to pay toward their college education, and many colleges understate living costs. This means that students in need of financial support—including those from moderate- and middle-income families—do not necessarily receive need-based grant aid to help pay for college.[12]

Relative to prior generations, today's undergraduates are more likely to have a job and to work longer hours, on average.[13] While students work for different reasons, it is clear that students from low-income and poor families work to pay for college and basic material goods, including food and shelter.[14] Unlike prior generations, however, twenty-first-century students cannot work their way through college with a combination of summer and part-time employment. Today, students would have to work a full-time job and a part-time job, year-round, in order to cover the costs of attending a public four-year college without going into debt.[15] Since the early 2000s, student employment has shifted into lower-wage jobs, including those in the service industry that tend to pay the minimum wage and lack a consistent or secure work schedule. After adjusting for inflation, the value of the federal minimum wage peaked 50 years ago. Indeed, since it was last raised to $7.25 per hour in 2009, it has lost 10 percent of its purchasing power to inflation.[16] Moreover, the median incomes of low- and middle-class families have stagnated since 2000, while upper-class families are earning more, widening income inequality in the United States.[17] Today, nearly one-third of adults live in a low-income household, with a median annual income of approximately $25,000 for a three-person household, and even more live in moderate-income households that struggle to make ends meet, yet they are ineligible for most public supports.[18]

These stagnant incomes, coupled with the rising net price of college, mean that students and their families must devote a larger share of their family income toward paying for college. After accounting for grant aid, more than half of undergraduates still face college prices greater than 25 percent of their family income. This includes both families that earn $60,000 per year but must pay more than $15,000 for college and families that earn $20,000 per year and must pay more than $5,000 out of pocket. Furthermore, 23 percent of today's undergraduates face net prices (full cost of attendance minus grant aid) that are equal to or exceed 100 percent of their total family income; in 2004, just 12 percent of students were asked to pay 100 percent or more of their total income toward college. In other words, the share of students whose families must devote all of their family income to pay for college has doubled over the past decade to one in four.[19]

Although rigorous research shows that additional financial resources improve degree attainment for students from low-income families, the current financial aid system leaves students short of financial security.[20] As noted above, most students work for pay, and some take out federal student loans, but the maximum amount often falls short of students' unmet need.[21] Students are left with few options: they can take out private loans, apply for additional scholarships, seek out public or private philanthropic resources, or stretch their budgets and cut back on basic material goods to try to make ends meet. It is against this backdrop that we examine the scope and depth of the problem of food insecurity in higher education.

Food Insecurity and Hunger on College Campuses

The best evidence indicates that approximately half of college undergraduates are food insecure, defined as limited or uncertain availability of nutritionally adequate and safe foods or ability to acquire such foods in a socially acceptable manner.[22] Although there are no nationally representative estimates of food insecurity among college students, a recent systematic review of the highest-quality studies found that 50.9 percent of college students are food insecure, after accounting for study sample size; when lower-quality studies were included in the analysis, the weighted mean was 47.2 percent.[23] Nationally, 12 percent of American households were food insecure in 2017, meaning they lacked access to enough food for an active, healthy life for all household members.[24] College students, therefore, appear to be at a much greater risk of food insecurity than the general public.

Food insecurity includes a range of experiences, and only the most severe are associated with the physiological sensation of hunger.[25] Based on the number of affirmative responses to a food security survey module, the US Department of Agriculture recognizes four categories of food security: high, marginal, low, and very low:[26]

- *High Food Security*: no reported food-access problems or limitations.
- *Marginal Food Security*: anxiety or worry over food sufficiency or food shortage, including concerns that food will not stretch to the end of the month or next paycheck.
- *Low Food Security*: reduced quality, variety, or desirability of diet, including substituting low-cost, lower-quality food items for higher-cost, higher-quality food items.
- *Very Low Food Security*: multiple indications of disrupted eating patterns and reduced food intake, including skipping or cutting the size of meals, which is often associated with hunger.

Though experiences of food insecurity and hunger affect all types of students attending colleges and universities in all sectors across the nation, some are at disproportionate risk.[27] Students from groups that have been historically and systemically marginalized are more likely to report experiences of food insecurity and hunger. In particular, students of color, LGBTQ students, former foster youth, first-generation college students, those from low-income families, and those with prior experiences of food insecurity are more likely to report food security challenges during college than their more advantaged peers.[28] Those with significant family responsibilities, including student parents, are also more likely to struggle with food insecurity. According to a recent survey from the Wisconsin HOPE Lab, the highest rates of food insecurity are among students who were ever in foster care (62% at two-year and 63% at four-year institutions), students who received the Pell Grant (55% at two-year and 46% at four-year institutions), black students (54% at two-year and 47% at four-year institutions), Native American students (55% at two-year and 30% at four-year institutions), multiracial students (50% at two-year and 42% at four-year institutions), bisexual students (54% at two-year and 47% at four-year institutions), gender nonbinary students (50% at two-year and 46% at four-year institutions), and student parents (52% at two-year and 43% at four-year institutions).[29]

Students who are food insecure describe an ongoing balancing act—one characterized by limited time and limited money—that often results in sacrificing food in the short term in hopes of longer-term socioeconomic success and stability associated with a college degree. When students do not have enough money to make ends meet, food is often the first thing to go: you have to eat every day, whereas other basic material goods like housing and clothing require less frequent purchases. To cope with food insecurity, some students eat cheap fast food or try to suppress hunger with excessive fluid intake. In prior studies, undergraduates have explained that they feel regretful for relying on "junk food" to feel full and have a preference for home-cooked meals, but they simply do not have the time or resources to eat more nutritious food.[30] Normalization of the "starving college student" trope and jokes about the "ramen noodle diet" as a rite of passage minimize students' very real food challenges and impede efforts to promote food security on college campuses.

Most students who are food insecure work and receive financial aid, but they still have trouble making ends meet given the high price of college and low wages.[31] There is even evidence that rates of food insecurity are higher among students who are employed or work long hours, likely because students who are struggling to make ends meet are searching for ways to earn more money.[32] In sharp contrast, a minority of students utilize food-related public assistance programs like SNAP owing to eligibility restrictions and barriers, stigma, and lack of awareness.[33] According to a 2018 report by the Government Accountability Office, less than half of students who were likely in need of and eligible for SNAP reported that they participated in the program.[34] The limited public social safety net is particularly consequential for students without a strong social and familial network to rely on for support.[35]

Implications for College Success and Student Well-Being

Strong theory and a growing body of research demonstrate that experiences of food insecurity and hunger during college are associated with poorer academic performance and attainment, physical and mental health, and well-being, undermining investments in higher education and impeding upward social mobility.[36] According to a longitudinal study of community college students, those who experience very low food security early in college are more than four percentage points less likely to graduate the following year, after accounting for differences in prior academic preparation and background characteristics.[37]

Scholars have studied food deprivation for well over a century, and the effects are well known: weight loss, physical illness, fatigue, irritability, decreased cognitive ability, and mental health problems, including depression.[38] However, one does not have to face starvation or experience *very low food security* for the ill effects of food insecurity to take hold. Lack of nutritious food (including those who have *low food security*) and chronic stress from worrying about your next meal (common among those with *marginal food security*) can also impede cognition and academic success.[39] When individuals are faced with near-term scarcity, they have less brainpower or cognitive bandwidth

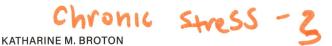

Chronic stress - 3

to devote to educational tasks, and the logistical challenges of relying on food pantries or obtaining and recertifying public benefits can take an incredible amount of time and patience.[40] Together, the reciprocal and reinforcing relationships between food insecurity and poor physical and mental health can create a negative feedback loop impeding students' ability to reach their full potential.[41]

Limitations and Next Steps

Though educators have long supported college students who are food insecure or struggle to meet the basic daily necessities of life, scholarly inquiry on basic needs insecurity in higher education is relatively recent, with almost all of the research occurring in just the past five years. This gap stands in sharp contrast to a clear focus in K–12 education research on how poverty and material hardship affect children's performance in school and on how policy efforts—such as the National School Lunch and Breakfast Programs and McKinney-Vento Homeless Education Assistance Act—try to ameliorate those conditions.[42]

Despite repeated requests by higher education scholars and practitioners, none of the nationally representative survey studies of college students conducted by the US Department of Education include a comprehensive measure of food insecurity.[43] Instead, the best evidence on the scope and depth of the problem comes from a series of multi-institutional studies, including those conducted by the Wisconsin HOPE Lab (now the Hope Center for College, Community, and Justice at Temple University), the University of California Global Food Initiative, and the California State University Basic Needs Initiative.[44] Though these studies employ best practices in survey research methodology, they lack the significant financial support needed to obtain representative estimates. Because students who are struggling to make ends meet may be less likely to participate in such studies, these estimates may actually be a conservative account of the problem.[45] Significant financial investment is necessary to obtain a nationally representative estimate of food insecurity among college students.

While national estimates of the problem are important to the development of national policy and programmatic responses, localized estimates are often the most useful in helping colleges and campuses take action. Since 2015, the Wisconsin HOPE Lab (now the Hope Center) has conducted an annual basic needs insecurity survey in which colleges and universities can participate to learn more about student experiences on their campus.[46] Countless other institutions have collaborated with local scholars or utilized their institutional research office to estimate the prevalence of food insecurity on their campus.[47]

However, we need to move beyond a definition of the problem in order to end hunger on college campuses. Food insecurity is a complex problem, and a more comprehensive understanding of the ways in which it manifests across contexts is necessary to fight it effectively. That means we need research and evaluation to determine the efficacy of programs and policies designed to promote food and basic needs security, and we also need to understand why and how an initiative works (or does not work), for whom, and under which conditions. Furthermore, the object of interest cannot be limited to students but must also include the ways in which those in power—including college, community, and policy leaders—perceive, understand, and support college students who experience basic needs insecurity.[48] These types of questions are difficult to answer; research that enables this sort of inquiry is often expensive and time-consuming, requiring cross-sector collaborations.[49] But we simply cannot afford the cost of inaction.

Conclusion

The current higher education system is failing too many of our students and communities.[50] Less than 10 percent of young adults from low-income families have a bachelor's degree even though nearly one-third have enrolled in college.[51] In fact, the gap in college completion rates between the rich and poor has grown in recent decades. Those from high-income families are now 45 percentage points, or roughly six times, more likely than those from low-income families to earn a bachelor's degree by age 25.[52] These gaps persist among the most academically prepared students and can be stemmed, at least in part, with additional financial resources.[53]

Approximately half of undergraduates—and especially those from historically marginalized and disadvantaged communities—report that they are struggling to meet basic daily necessities like adequate food, and such material hardships are impeding their academic success. There is no evidence that the share of students experiencing basic needs insecurity has improved in recent years, and the increasing net price of college attendance will likely only exacerbate the problem.[54] Something must be done. This book contains the latest promising practices designed to promote basic needs security so that students can learn and reach their educational and life goals. Research in collaboration with practitioners and policymakers can help us understand whether these initiatives are working and the best ways to reach our common goals.

A college credential pays dividends—not only for the individual with a well-paying job but also for the communities in which they are civically involved and the health of our nation more broadly.[55] These social returns often exceed private ones, and the benefits of a college degree are largest among those least likely to attain one.[56] Disproportionate college completion rates inhibit efforts to create an educated workforce and citizenry, as well as a more socially equitable society.[57] Beyond an individual human right to food, improving food security can enhance the health, well-being, and educational success of students and our communities.[58]

Notes

1. All names have been changed.
2. To learn more about the meal voucher program and related study, see Sara Goldrick-Rab, Katharine M. Broton, and Daphne C. Hernandez,

Addressing Basic Needs Security in Higher Education: An Introduction to Three Evaluations of Supports for Food and Housing at Community Colleges (Madison: Wisconsin HOPE Lab, 2017), https://hope4college.com/wp -content/uploads/2018/09/Addressing-Basic-Needs-Security-in-Higher -Education.pdf.

3. Anne-Marie Hamelin, Micheline Beaudry, and Jean-Pierre Habicht, "Characterization of Household Food Insecurity in Québec: Food and Feelings," *Social Science and Medicine* 54, no. 1 (Jan. 2002): 119–32, https:// doi.org/10.1016/S0277-9536(01)00013-2; Kathy L. Radimer, Christine M. Olson, and Cathy C. Campbell, "Development of Indicators to Assess Hunger," *Journal of Nutrition* 120, no. S11 (1990): 1544–48, https://doi.org /10.1093/jn/120.suppl_11.1544.

4. See, e.g., Pam Y. Eddinger, "Food for Thought: How Building a Hunger Team on Campus Helped BHCC Advocate for the Basic Needs of Its Students," *Bunker Hill Community College Magazine* 13, no. 1 (Spring 2017), https://www.bhcc.edu/magazine/pastissues/BHCCMagazine_June2017.pdf.

5. "Adult BMI Calculator," Center for Disease Control, https://www.cdc .gov/healthyweight/assessing/bmi/adult_bmi/english_bmi_calculator/bmi _calculator.html.

6. US Department of Education, *Demographic and Enrollment Characteristics of Nontraditional Undergraduates: 2011–12* (Washington, DC: US Department of Education, Sept. 2015), https://nces.ed.gov/pubs2015 /2015025.pdf.

7. US Department of Education, *Demographic and Enrollment Characteristics.*

8. Author's calculations based on "National Postsecondary Student Aid Study (NPSAS): 2016," National Center for Education Statistics, https://nces .ed.gov/surveys/npsas/.

9. College Board, *Trends in College Pricing* (New York: College Board, 2017), https://trends.collegeboard.org/sites/default/files/2017-trends-in -college-pricing_1.pdf.

10. Author's calculations based on "National Postsecondary Student Aid Study (NPSAS): 2016."

11. Sara Goldrick-Rab, *Paying the Price: College Costs, Financial Aid, and the Betrayal of the American Dream* (Chicago: University of Chicago Press, 2016).

12. Robert Kelchen, Sara Goldrick-Rab, and Braden Hosch, "The Costs of College Attendance: Examining Variation and Consistency in Institutional Living Cost Allowances," *Journal of Higher Education* 88, no. 6 (2017): 947–71, https://doi.org/10.1080/00221546.2016.1272092. Moreover, students who do not receive any financial support from their families do not necessarily meet the requirements to be declared "financially independent" by the financial aid system; Goldrick-Rab, *Paying the Price.*

13. Judith Scott-Clayton, "What Explains Trends in Labor Supply among US Undergraduates?," *National Tax Journal* 65, no. 1 (2012): 181–210, https://doi.org/10.17310/ntj.2012.1.07.

14. Katharine M. Broton, Sara Goldrick-Rab, and James Benson, "Working for College: The Causal Impacts of Financial Grants on Undergraduate Employment," *Educational Evaluation and Policy Analysis* 38, no. 3 (2016): 477–94, https://doi.org/10.3102/0162373716638440.

15. Judith Scott-Clayton, "The Causal Effect of Federal Work-Study Participation: Quasi-experimental Evidence from West Virginia," *Educational Evaluation and Policy Analysis* 33, no. 4 (2011): 506–27, https://doi.org/10.3102/0162373711421211.

16. The share of employed full-time undergraduates working in the service industry went from approximately 20% in 1970 to 35% in 2009. Over the same time period, the share of students working in the professional, technical, managerial, and clerical sector declined from roughly 45% to 30%; Scott-Clayton, "What Explains Trends." For information on the minimum wage and the nature of work, see Drew Desilver, *Five Facts about the Minimum Wage* (Washington, DC: Pew Research Center, Jan. 4, 2017), http://www.pewresearch.org/fact-tank/2017/01/04/5-facts-about-the-minimum-wage/; Arne L. Kalleberg, *Good Jobs, Bad Jobs: The Rise of Polarized and Precarious Employment Systems in the United States, 1970s to 2000s* (New York: Russell Sage Foundation, 2011); Susan J. Lambert, Peter J. Fugiel, and Julia R. Henly, *Precarious Work Schedules among Early-Career Employees in the US: A National Snapshot* (Chicago: Employment Instability, Family Well-Being, and Social Policy Network at the University of Chicago, 2014), https://ssa.uchicago.edu/sites/default/files/uploads/lambert.fugiel.henly_.precarious_work_schedules.august2014_0.pdf.

17. Rakesh Kochhar, *The American Middle Class Is Stable in Size, but Losing Ground Financially to Upper-Income Families* (Washington, DC: Pew Research Center, Sept. 6, 2018), http://www.pewresearch.org/fact-tank/2018/09/06/the-american-middle-class-is-stable-in-size-but-losing-ground-financially-to-upper-income-families/.

18. Kochhar, *American Middle Class.*

19. Robert Kelchen, "Trends in Net Prices by Family Income," *Kelchen on Education* (blog), June 6, 2018, https://robertkelchen.com/kelchen-on-education/. Author's calculations based on "National Postsecondary Student Aid Study (NPSAS): 2016."

20. Benjamin L. Castleman and Bridget Terry Long, "Looking beyond Enrollment: The Causal Effect of Need-Based Grants on College Access, Persistence, and Graduation," *Journal of Labor Economics* 34, no. 4 (2016): 1023–73, https://doi.org/10.1086/686643; Sara Goldrick-Rab et al., "Reducing Income Inequality in Educational Attainment: Experimental Evidence on the Impact of Financial Aid on College Completion," *American Journal of Sociology* 121, no. 6 (2016): 1762–1817, https://doi.org/10.1086/685442.

21. For first-year dependent students, federal financial loans are capped at $5,500, and only $3,500 can be subsidized. The maximum allowance increases to $6,500 and $7,500 in later years, with a career maximum of $31,000; Goldrick-Rab, *Paying the Price.*

22. The best evidence on the prevalence of food insecurity among undergraduates comes from multi-institutional and statewide studies of undergraduates rather than studies of students at a single institution or studies of households, which do not necessarily accurately reflect the daily realities of college students who may be living apart from their family. See Katharine M. Broton and Sara Goldrick-Rab, "Going Without: An Exploration of Food and Housing Insecurity among Undergraduates," *Educational Researcher* 47, no. 2 (2018): 121–33, https://doi.org/10.3102 /0013189X17741303; Rashida Crutchfield and Jennifer Maguire, *Study of Student Basic Needs* (Long Beach: California State University, Office of the Chancellor, Jan. 2018), https://www2.calstate.edu/impact-of-the-csu /student-success/basic-needs-initiative/Documents/BasicNeedsStudy _phaseII_withAccessibilityComments.pdf; Nicholas Freudenberg et al., *Food Insecurity at CUNY: Results from a Survey of CUNY Undergraduate Students* (New York: Campaign for a Healthy CUNY, 2011), https://www.gc .cuny.edu/CUNY_GC/media/CUNY-Graduate-Center/PDF/Centers /Center%20for%20Human%20Environments/cunyfoodinsecurity.pdf; Suzanna M. Martinez, Katie Maynard, and Lorrene D. Ritchie, *Student Food Access and Security Study* (University of California Global Food Initiative, Office of the President, 2016), https://regents.universityofcalifornia.edu /regmeet/july16/e1attach.pdf. According to a 2018 Government Accountability Office (GAO) report, just eight of the thirty-one studies included in their review included survey respondents from multiple college campuses; US Government Accountability Office, *Food Insecurity: Better Information Could Help Eligible College Students Access Federal Food Assistance Benefits* (Washington, DC: US Government Accountability Office [GAO-19-95], Published Dec. 2018 and Publicly Released Jan. 2019), https://www.gao.gov /products/GAO-19-95, 12. Most of the studies they reviewed (22 of 31), however, estimated student food insecurity prevalence rates over 30%, with many clustering around half. Some of the studies included in the 2018 GAO review were not designed to measure the prevalence of food insecurity among college students and only include a subpopulation of all undergraduates. For example, Gaines, Robb, Knol, and Sickler only include full-time, returning students who are 19–25 years old and not pregnant in their study of the relationship among financial factors, resources and skills, and food security status because their goal was to capture the "traditional college experience"; Alisha Gaines et al., "Examining the Role of Financial Factors, Resources and Skills in Predicting Food Security Status among College Students: Food Security and Resource Adequacy," *International Journal of Consumer Studies* 38, no. 4 (2014): 374–84, 377, https://doi.org/10.1111/ijcs .12110. This single institution study is located in an area that was "recently affected by a significant natural disaster" (374). The authors report that 14% of survey respondents have low or very low levels of food security (i.e., on par with national household estimates), but the sample excludes many vulnerable students who are likely at greater risk of food insecurity (e.g., part-time students, those who were not retained into the second year of

college, pregnant students, and those displaced by a natural disaster). This is almost certainly a conservative estimate of the problem, as it is not representative of the roughly three-quarters of undergraduates who do not have a "traditional college experience" and are at greater risk of food insecurity (US Government Accountability Office, *Food Insecurity*). Food insecurity is defined in accordance with Sue Ann Anderson, "Core Indicators of Nutritional State for Difficult-to-Sample Populations," *Journal of Nutrition* 120, no. S11 (1990): 1555–1600, https://doi.org/10.1093/jn/120.suppl_11.1555.

23. Aydin Nazmi et al., "A Systematic Review of Food Insecurity among US Students in Higher Education," *Journal of Hunger and Environmental Nutrition* 13, no. 1 (2018): 1–16, https://doi.org/10.1080/19320248.2018.1484316.

24. Alisha Coleman-Jensen et al., *Household Food Security in the United States in 2017* (Washington, DC: US Department of Agriculture Economic Research Service, Sept. 2018), https://www.ers.usda.gov/publications/pub-details/?pubid=90022.

25. Katharine M. Broton, Kari E. Weaver, and Minhtuyen Mai, "Hunger in Higher Education: Experiences and Correlates of Food Insecurity among Wisconsin Undergraduates from Low-Income Families," *Social Sciences* 7, no. 10 (2018): 179, https://doi.org/10.3390/socsci7100179; Lisa Henry, "Understanding Food Insecurity among College Students: Experience, Motivation, and Local Solutions," *Annals of Anthropological Practice* 41, no. 1 (2017): 6–19, https://doi.org/doi:10.1111/napa.12108.

26. For a brief history and measurement overview of food insecurity in the United States, see Gary Bickel et al., *Guide to Measuring Household Food Security*, rev. ed. (Alexandria, VA: US Department of Agriculture, Food and Nutrition Service, Office of Analysis, Nutrition, and Evaluation, 2000), https://www.fns.usda.gov/guide-measuring-household-food-security-revised-2000; Katharine M. Broton, "The Evolution of Poverty in Higher Education: Material Hardship, Academic Success, and Policy Perspectives" (PhD diss., University of Wisconsin–Madison, 2017), appendix A; National Research Council, Panel to Review US Department of Agriculture's Measurement of Food Insecurity and Hunger, Committee on National Statistics, and Division of Behavioral and Social Sciences and Education, *Measuring Food Insecurity and Hunger: Phase 1 Report* (Washington, DC: National Academies Press, 2005), https://www.nap.edu/catalog/11227/measuring-food-insecurity-and-hunger-phase-1-report; Tammy Ouellette et al., *Measures of Material Hardship: Final Report* (Washington, DC: US Department of Health and Human Services, Office of the Assistant Secretary for Planning and Evaluation, 2004), https://aspe.hhs.gov/report/measures-material-hardship-final-report.

27. Though the majority of the research has been on public two- and four-year institutions, there is also evidence of food insecurity in the private college sector. See, e.g., Cara Cliburn Allen and Nathan Alleman, "A Private Struggle at a Private Institution: Effects of Student Hunger on Social and Academic Experiences," *Journal of College Student Development* 60, no. 1

(2019): 52–69; Anthony A. Jack, "'I, Too, Am Hungry': An Examination of Structural Exclusion at an Elite University" (invited presentation, University of Wisconsin–Madison, Apr. 24, 2015).

28. Broton, Weaver, and Mai, "Hunger in Higher Education"; Clare L. Cady, "Food Insecurity as a Student Issue," *Journal of College and Character* 15, no. 4 (2014): 265-72, https://doi.org/10.1515/jcc-2014-0031; Sara Goldrick-Rab et al., *Still Hungry and Homeless in College* (Madison: Wisconsin HOPE Lab, 2018), https://hope4college.com/wp-content/uploads/2018/09/Wisconsin-HOPE-Lab-Still-Hungry-and-Homeless.pdf; Suzanna M. Martinez et al., "Food Insecurity in California's Public University System: What Are the Risk Factors?," *Journal of Hunger and Environmental Nutrition* 13, no. 1 (2018): 1–18, https://doi.org/10.1080/19320248.2017.1374901; Nazmi et al., "Systematic Review of Food Insecurity"; Devon C. Payne-Sturges et al., "Student Hunger on Campus: Food Insecurity among College Students and Implications for Academic Institutions," *American Journal of Health Promotion* 32, no. 2 (2018): 349-54, https://doi.org/10.1177/0890117117719620.

29. Goldrick-Rab et al., *Still Hungry and Homeless in College.*

30. Broton, Weaver, and Mai, "Hunger in Higher Education"; Henry, "Understanding Food Insecurity."

31. Broton and Goldrick-Rab, "Going Without."

32. Freudenberg et al., *Food Insecurity at CUNY*; Goldrick-Rab et al., *Still Hungry and Homeless in College*; Megan M. Patton-López et al., "Prevalence and Correlates of Food Insecurity among Students Attending a Midsize Rural University in Oregon," *Journal of Nutrition Education and Behavior* 46, no. 3 (May 1, 2014): 209-14, https://doi.org/10.1016/j.jneb.2013.10.007.

33. Broton and Goldrick-Rab, "Going Without"; Amy Ellen Duke-Benfield, *Bolstering Non-traditional Student Success: A Comprehensive Student Aid System Using Financial Aid, Public Benefits, and Refundable Tax Credits* (Washington, DC: Center for Postsecondary and Economic Success, 2015), https://www.clasp.org/sites/default/files/public/resources-and-publications/publication-1/Bolstering-NonTraditional-Student-Success.pdf.

34. US Government Accountability Office, *Food Insecurity.*

35. Broton, Weaver, and Mai, "Hunger in Higher Education."

36. In higher education, see, e.g., Broton, "Evolution of Poverty"; Daniel Eisenberg et al., *Too Distressed to Learn? Mental Health among Community College Students* (Madison: Wisconsin HOPE Lab, 2016), https://hope4college.com/wp-content/uploads/2018/09/Wisconsin_HOPE_Lab-Too_Distressed_To_Learn.pdf; Freudenberg et al., *Food Insecurity at CUNY*; Goldrick-Rab et al., *Still Hungry and Homeless in College*; Maya E. Maroto, Anastasia Snelling, and Henry Linck, "Food Insecurity among Community College Students: Prevalence and Association with Grade Point Average," *Community College Journal of Research and Practice* 39, no. 6 (June 3, 2015): 515-26; Martinez et al., "Food Insecurity in California's Public University System"; Loran Mary Morris et al., "The Prevalence of Food Security and

Insecurity among Illinois University Students," *Journal of Nutrition Education and Behavior* 48, no. 6 (June 1, 2016): 376-82.e1, https://doi.org/10.1016 /j.jneb.2016.03.013; Patton-López et al., "Prevalence and Correlates of Food Insecurity"; Erica Phillips, Anne McDaniel, and Alicia Croft, "Food Insecurity and Academic Disruption among College Students," *Journal of Student Affairs Research and Practice* 55, no. 4 (Oct. 2, 2018): 353-72, https:// doi.org/10.1080/19496591.2018.1470003; Irene van Woerden, Daniel Hruschka, and Meg Bruening, "Food Insecurity Negatively Impacts Academic Performance," *Journal of Public Affairs*, Nov. 26, 2018, e1864, https://doi.org/10.1002/pa.1864. In addition, studies on K–12 children also demonstrate a relationship. See, e.g., Katherine Alaimo, "Food Insecurity in the United States: An Overview," *Topics in Clinical Nutrition* 20, no. 4 (2005): 281-98, https://doi.org/10.1097/00008486-200510000-00002; Diana F. Jyoti, Edward A. Frongillo, and Sonya J. Jones, "Food Insecurity Affects School Children's Academic Performance, Weight Gain, and Social Skills," *Journal of Nutrition* 135 no. 12 (2005): 2831-39, https://doi.org/10.1093/jn/135 .12.2831; Joshua Winicki and Kyle Jemison, "Food Insecurity and Hunger in the Kindergarten Classroom: Its Effect on Learning and Growth," *Contemporary Economic Policy* 21, no. 2 (Apr. 1, 2003): 145-57, https://doi.org /doi:10.1093/cep/byg001.

37. Katharine M. Broton, "How Hunger and Homelessness Affect Community College Students' Academic Achievement and Attainment" (lecture, American Educational Association Annual Meeting, New York, NY, 2018).

38. See, e.g., The Minnesota Starvation Experiment (1944–45) and related research, including David Baker and Natacha Keramidas, "The Psychology of Hunger," *Monitor on Psychology* 44, no. 9 (Oct. 2013), https://www.apa .org/monitor/2013/10/hunger.aspx; Ancel Keys et al., *The Biology of Human Starvation*, 2 vols. (Minneapolis: University of Minnesota Press, 1950); Todd Tucker, *The Great Starvation Experiment: Ancel Keys and the Men Who Starved for Science* (Minneapolis: University of Minnesota Press, 2007). For a nineteenth-century study, see, e.g., D. Noël Paton and Ralph Stockman, "Observations on the Metabolism of Man during Starvation," *Proceedings of the Royal Society of Edinburgh* 16 (1890): 121–31.

39. Broton, "Evolution of Poverty"; John T. Cook and Deborah A. Frank, "Food Security, Poverty, and Human Development in the United States," *Annals of the New York Academy of Sciences* 1136, no. 1 (2008): 193-209, https://doi.org/10.1196/annals.1425.001; Fernando Gómez-Pinilla, "Brain Foods: The Effects of Nutrients on Brain Function," *Nature Reviews Neuroscience* 9, no. 7 (2008): 568-78, https://doi.org/10.1038/nrn2421; Jill S. Halterman et al., "Iron Deficiency and Cognitive Achievement among School-Aged Children and Adolescents in the United States," *Pediatrics* 107, no. 6 (2001): 1381-86; Sonia J. Lupien et al., "Effects of Stress throughout the Lifespan on the Brain, Behaviour and Cognition," *Nature Reviews Neuroscience* 10, no. 6 (2009): 434-45, https://doi.org/10.1038/nrn2639.

40. Katharine M. Broton and Sara Goldrick-Rab, "The Dark Side of College (Un)Affordability: Food and Housing Insecurity in Higher Education,"

Change Magazine 48, no. 1 (2016): 16–25, https://doi.org/10.1080/00091383 .2016.1121081; Sendhil Mullainathan and Eldar Shafir, *Scarcity: Why Having Too Little Means So Much* (New York: Times Books, 2013).

41. David M. Cutler and Adriana Lleras-Muney, "Education and Health: Evaluating Theories and Evidence" (working paper no. w12352, National Bureau of Economic Research, 2006); Eisenberg et al., *Too Distressed to Learn?*

42. See, e.g., Alaimo, "Food Insecurity in the United States"; Sidse S. Andersen, Lotte Holm, and Charlotte Baarts, "School Meal Sociality or Lunch Pack Individualism? Using an Intervention Study to Compare the Social Impacts of School Meals and Packed Lunches from Home," *Social Science Information* 54, no. 3 (2015): 394–416, https://doi.org/10.1177 /0539018415584697; Dorothy Blair, "The Child in the Garden: An Evaluative Review of the Benefits of School Gardening," *Journal of Environmental Education* 40, no. 2 (2009): 15–38, https://doi.org/10.3200/JOEE.40.2.15-38; David E. Frisvold, "Nutrition and Cognitive Achievement: An Evaluation of the School Breakfast Program," *Journal of Public Economics* 124 (2015): 91–104, https://doi.org/10.1016/j.jpubeco.2014.12.003; Patricia Constante Jaime and Karen Lock, "Do School Based Food and Nutrition Policies Improve Diet and Reduce Obesity?," *Preventive Medicine* 48, no. 1 (2009): 45–53, https://doi.org/10.1016/j.ypmed.2008.10.018; Jyoti, Frongillo, and Jones, "Food Insecurity Affects School Children's Academic Performance"; Kathy L. Radimer et al., "Understanding Hunger and Developing Indicators to Assess It in Women and Children," *Journal of Nutrition Education* 24, no. 1 (1992): 36S–44S, https://doi.org/10.1016/S0022-3182(12)80137-3; Wendy J. Wills et al., "The Socio-economic Boundaries Shaping Young People's Lunchtime Food Practices on a School Day," *Children and Society* 32, no. 3 (2018): 195–206, https://doi.org/10.1111/chso.12261; Winicki and Jemison, "Food Insecurity and Hunger." For an exception, see Sara Goldrick-Rab, Katharine M. Broton, and Emily Brunjes Colo, *Why the Time Is Right to Expand the National School Lunch Program to Higher Education* (Scholars Strategy Network, 2016), https://scholars.org/brief/why-time-right-expand -national-school-lunch-program-higher-education.

43. Wisconsin HOPE Lab and American Council on Education Center for Policy Research and Strategy, *Request to Add Measurement of Food Insecurity to the National Postsecondary Student Aid Study* (Madison: Wisconsin HOPE Lab, 2015), https://hope4college.com/wp-content/uploads/2018/09 /NPSAS-Brief-2015_WI-HOPE-Lab_ACE.pdf. A recent article by Lois Elfman, however, reports that Kathryn Larin, director of the Education, Workforce, and Income Security Team at the Government Accountability Office, recently indicated that "there is a plan by the National Postsecondary Student Aid Study (NPSAS) to start including questions related to food insecurity"; Lois Elfman, "GAO Report Tackles Issues of Food Insecurity among College Students," *Diverse Issues in Higher Education*, Jan. 9, 2019, https://diverseeducation.com/article/135731/.

44. Broton and Goldrick-Rab, "Going Without"; Crutchfield and Maguire, *Study of Student Basic Needs*; Freudenberg et al., *Food Insecurity at*

CUNY; Goldrick-Rab et al., *Still Hungry and Homeless in College*; Sara Goldrick-Rab, Jed Richardson, and Anthony Hernandez, *Hungry and Homeless in College: Results from a National Study of Basic Needs Insecurity in Higher Education* (Madison: Wisconsin HOPE Lab, 2017), https:// hope4college.com/wp-content/uploads/2018/09/Hungry-and-Homeless-in -College-Report.pdf; Sara Goldrick-Rab, Katharine Broton, and Daniel Eisenberg, *Hungry to Learn: Addressing Food and Housing Insecurity among Undergraduates* (Madison: Wisconsin HOPE Lab, Dec. 2015), https:// hope4college.com/wp-content/uploads/2018/09/Wisconsin_HOPE_Lab _Hungry_To_Learn.pdf; Martinez, Maynard, and Ritchie, *Student Food Access and Security Study*.

45. Katharine M. Broton et al., "Who's Hungry? Making Sense of Campus Food Insecurity Estimates," *Medium* (blog), Jan. 22, 2018, https://medium .com/@saragoldrickrab/whos-hungry-making-sense-of-campus-food -insecurity-estimates-4b65cd1ecf2c; Sara Goldrick-Rab and Katharine M. Broton, "On Estimating Food Insecurity among Undergraduates," *Medium* (blog), Aug. 1, 2017, https://medium.com/@saragoldrickrab/on-estimating -food-insecurity-among-undergraduates-a7db0cf79632; Goldrick-Rab et al., *Still Hungry and Homeless in College*.

46. See Hope Center for College, Community, and Justice's #RealCollege Survey website, https://realcollege.org/realcollege-survey/, for more information; see also *Real College: A Study of the Real Experiences of College Students* (Philadelphia: Hope Center for College, Community, and Justice), https://drive.google.com/file/d/1RplSIrNUO9OyoBzVSsstjAm4zkZDeDhz /view.

47. This is how much of the research on food insecurity on college campuses started. See, e.g., M. Pia Chaparro et al., "Food Insecurity Prevalence among College Students at the University of Hawai'i at Mānoa," *Public Health Nutrition* 12, no. 11 (2009): 2097–103, https://doi.org /10.1017/S1368980009990735.

48. See, e.g., Katharine M. Broton, Graham N. S. Miller, and Sara Goldrick-Rab, "College on the Margins: Higher Education Professionals' Perspectives on Campus Basic Needs Insecurity," *Teachers College Record* (forthcoming).

49. For examples of mixed-methods longitudinal research studies that involve cross-sector collaborations, see Goldrick-Rab, Broton, and Hernandez, *Addressing Basic Needs Security*; Derek Price et al., *Public Benefits and Community Colleges: Lessons from the Benefits Access for College Completion Evaluation* (Philadelphia: OMG Center for Collaborative Learning, 2014), http://www.equalmeasure.org/wp-content/uploads/2014/12/BACC-Final -Report-FINAL-111914.pdf.

50. Goldrick-Rab, *Paying the Price*.

51. Kathleen M. Ziol-Guest and Kenneth T. H. Lee, "Parent Income–Based Gaps in Schooling: Cross-Cohort Trends in the NLSYs and the PSID," *AERA Open* 2, no. 2 (Apr. 1, 2016): 1–10, https://doi.org/10.1177 /2332858416645834.

52. Martha J. Bailey and Susan M. Dynarski, "Gains and Gaps: Changing Inequality in U.S. College Entry and Completion" (working paper no. 17633, National Bureau of Economic Research, Dec. 2011), https://www.nber.org/papers/w17633.pdf; Ziol-Guest and Lee, "Parent Income–Based Gaps in Schooling."

53. Castleman and Long, "Looking beyond Enrollment"; Goldrick-Rab et al., "Reducing Income Inequality"; National Center for Education Statistics, *Condition of Education* (Washington, DC: US Department of Education, 2015).

54. Broton and Goldrick-Rab, "Going Without."

55. Clive R. Belfield and Thomas Bailey, "The Benefits of Attending Community College: A Review of the Evidence," *Community College Review* 39, no. 1 (2011): 46–68, https://doi.org/10.1177/0091552110395575; Philip Oreopoulos and Uros Petronijevic, "Making College Worth It: A Review of the Returns to Higher Education," *Future of Children* 23, no. 1 (2013): 41–65.

56. Michael Hout, "Social and Economic Returns to College Education in the United States," *Annual Review of Sociology* 38, no. 1 (2012): 379–400, https://doi.org/10.1146/annurev.soc.012809.102503.

57. Anthony P. Carnevale, Nicole Smith, and Jeff Strohl, *Help Wanted: Projections of Job and Education Requirements through 2018* (Washington, DC: Georgetown University Center on Education and the Workforce, 2010), https://cew.georgetown.edu/cew-reports/help-wanted/; Robert Haveman and Timothy Smeeding, "The Role of Higher Education in Social Mobility," *Future of Children* 16, no. 2 (2006): 125–50; National Center for Education Statistics, *Digest of Education Statistics* (Washington, DC: US Department of Education, 2013), https://nces.ed.gov/pubsearch/pubsinfo.asp?pubid=2015011; US Department of Education, *Meeting the Nation's 2020 Goal: State Targets for Increasing the Number and Percentage of College Graduates with Degrees* (Washington, DC: US Department of Education, 2011), https://www2.ed.gov/policy/highered/guid/secletter/110323insert.pdf.

58. Yasmine Dominguez-Whitehead, "Conceptualising Food Research in Higher Education as a Matter of Social Justice: Philosophical, Methodological and Ethical Considerations," *Cambridge Journal of Education* 47, no. 4 (2017): 551–65, https://doi.org/10.1080/0305764X.2016.1216087; Price et al., *Public Benefits and Community Colleges*; United Nations Centre for Human Rights, *Right to Adequate Food as a Human Right* (New York: United Nations, 1989); United Nations General Assembly, *Universal Declaration of Human Rights* (New York: United Nations General Assembly, 1948).

[2]

If Not Us, Who?

Building National Capacity to Address Student
Food Insecurity through CUFBA

CLARE L. CADY

Editors' Prologue. Keenly aware that college students experience hunger and
food insecurity, higher education administrators, faculty, staff, and students
have designed and implemented programs to address this issue and promote
student success.[1] The campus food pantry is the most common among these
approaches, with many colleges seeking out opportunities to learn from
others about pantry models and success strategies. When the College and
University Food Bank Alliance (CUFBA) was formed, there were a lot of
questions and very few people who could answer them. This chapter provides
a historical overview of the organization, discusses common ways that
colleges develop their campus pantries, and includes recommendations on
ways to implement and effectively manage a campus pantry. A capacity-
building organization, CUFBA provides much-needed education and
support to the growing and developing movement to address food insecurity
among students.

About the Author. Clare L. Cady (she/her/hers) served for seven years as
founding director of the College and University Food Bank Alliance and is a
scholar-practitioner working in the intersection of higher education and
human services. She has supported hundreds of colleges and universities in
developing programs to address basic needs insecurities among students.
Her work has been published in the *Journal of College and Character* and
About Campus and has been featured on NPR and MSNBC. She is a consultant,

writer, and public speaker on the issue of basic needs insecurities among college students.

The College and University Food Bank Alliance (CUFBA) was launched to forge collegial connections among practitioners engaging in human services work on college campuses, with an emphasis on the most common initiative seeking to address food insecurity—the campus food pantry. In 2011, cofounders Nate Smith-Tyge and I were practitioners managing programs addressing student hunger. At Michigan State University (MSU), Nate managed one of the oldest campus pantries in the county, the MSU Student Food Bank, serving thousands of pounds of food annually. I was overseeing the work of the Human Services Resource Center (HSRC) at Oregon State University (OSU), a student fee–funded office focused on alleviating poverty, hunger, and homelessness among students at OSU. At the time, there were few pantries on college campuses, and the literature on student food insecurity was limited to two studies.[2] Both Nate and I felt we lacked the support on campus or in existing professional networks to identify and utilize best practices and assess and improve our programs. Each of us went online to seek professionals doing similar work across the country, finding one another and bonding around this shared goal.

Harnessing my higher education background and Nate's focus on organizational studies, we developed a strategic plan to launch a professional organization focused on the management of campus food pantries. Pooling lists of programs we had already identified, we recruited practitioners from 15 colleges and universities to join the network. A year later, we launched a website and announced a grand opening, presenting our work and CUFBA's mission and goals at the 2012 National Association of Student Personnel Administrators conference for student affairs professionals. At the conference, we actively recruited colleges and universities with campus pantries to join the network. We also learned that although very few colleges had campus pantries, many were eager to learn more about this intervention to address food insecurity among their students.

As awareness of food insecurity among students grew, more colleges and universities began seeking models for programs that would address the issue. While Nate and I had launched CUFBA to engage in reciprocal learning opportunities and help improve our programs, the CUFBA website, overwhelmingly, generated requests for assistance in designing and launching *new* campus food pantries. Students, faculty, and administrators on college campuses, as well as members of the press, reached out to me and Nate after finding CUFBA online. By the start of the 2013–14 school year, we were fielding 8–10 inquiries per week, providing detailed accounts of how our programs worked, where we got our funding, and ways to get hesitant campus leadership to take the issue of food insecurity among students seriously.

Often upon the request of a champion who wanted to start a campus pantry, Nate and I found ourselves hosting conference calls with campus leadership and other stakeholders. During these calls, we dealt with skepticism from campus leaders who questioned whether the issue was prevalent enough to warrant resources dedicated to a new program or intervention; we heard statements such as "I ate ramen and beans in college and I made it through" and "Sure this might be an issue, but we are not social workers. This is not our responsibility to fix." Despite reticence and criticism, Nate and I made a case for why food insecurity was a student issue that needed to be addressed, and we saw the number of campuses starting food pantries grow. Reporters also took note of the issue. Media calls became so common for me that OSU requested I take public relations training. At one point, the external affairs office told me that I was getting more media inquiries than the college president.

The requests and attention pressed Nate and I to evaluate the assumptions we had made about the gap in the field. Though there was, indeed, a gap in professional connection around campus pantries, our approach was not filling that gap appropriately. The needs of our colleagues were much larger than anticipated, and there were even fewer people doing hunger relief work on campuses than we had imagined. We concluded that what was needed in the field was not collegial connection but teachers—we had to *create* the colleagues before we could *connect* with them. We rewrote CUFBA's strategic plan, changing its goals from reactively bringing together people who were already doing the work to proactively supporting the creation of new programs across the country.

Despite this shift in mission and goals, CUFBA maintained the guiding principle that students are better served when campus communities collaborate and communicate. We began to connect campuses within the same geographies or with similar characteristics so they could learn from one another. We systematized recruiting, supporting, and developing campus pantry programs, adding new team members as the network grew from 15 to over 500 in just four years. Such exponential growth was the result of intentional outreach, effective use of internet branding, never turning down media requests (no matter how small the outlet), and the willingness to be responsive to the needs of the field. At the time of writing this chapter, CUFBA's membership has topped 700 campuses and continues to grow.

CUFBA seeks to evolve to stay on the growth edge, maximize efficiencies, and take the work of addressing student hunger to scale. In 2014, providing individualized one-on-one consulting for all new members became unmanageable owing to high demand. The CUFBA team addressed this issue by designing toolkits and additional web-based resources to help programs get started, saving our higher-touch work for troubleshooting and capacity building rather than providing one-on-one support for startups. The first toolkit was developed by a graduate student at the University of Arkansas, Brandon Mathews, who later joined the CUFBA team as an associate director. In 2015, CUFBA partnered with the Student Government Resource Center to create an additional toolkit aimed at student leaders.[3] As interest in the issue of student food insecurity grew,

CUFBA leaders expanded their offerings to include presentations and trainings, traveling to conferences and convenings and scaling their teachings to reach multiple institutions at one time. This included having a presence as a leader in the field at the first #RealCollege Convening, an annual conference on basic needs insecurities among college students.

In 2014, CUFBA began to develop a metanetwork of other organizations addressing student hunger, including Swipe Out Hunger, Campus Kitchens Project, and the Food Recovery Network. The goal of this network is to increase the capacity of all organizations by collaborating and sharing lessons learned and resources. Additionally, the goal for these organizations is to engage in ongoing referrals to one another when working with colleges, avoiding mission creep by connecting campuses with experts in each area (food swipe donations, food recovery, etc.) rather than trying to duplicate services in areas where the referring organization was not as strong. More recently, CUFBA partnered with the National Student Campaign Against Hunger and Homelessness and Student PIRGs (Public Interest Research Groups) to administer a field survey of food insecurity on over 34 college and university campuses.[4] This report, published in 2016, aligned with other research in the field conducted at community colleges,[5] providing further evidence that food insecurity is a prevalent and problematic issue on college campuses. While this foray into research was a positive experience, CUFBA made the decision to collaborate again with organizations that have more expertise in a specific area through a partnership with the Hope Center for College, Community, and Justice, producing a report on campus pantry implementation that will be discussed later in this chapter.

As programs to address student hunger move beyond the campus pantry, CUFBA has sought to use the lessons learned from its work to help campus members take a more multifaceted approach to their work. In the 2016–17 academic year, CUFBA expanded its strategic plan to include all initiatives focused on student hunger, and it forged strong partnerships with others seeking to address students' basic needs in a multifaceted manner, such as the Hope Center for College, Community, and Justice at Temple University and the University of California's Global Food Initiative.

Strategies for Campus Pantries

CUFBA plays a powerful role in helping to shape the work of colleges and universities across the country, providing no-cost phone and email consultation, digital resources, and periodic workshops and presentations focused on helping college faculty, staff, and students understand food insecurity on campuses and how a campus pantry could help alleviate it. Although an on-campus food pantry for students is not required, CUFBA members must be engaged in work to alleviate student food insecurity. CUFBA charges no membership fees and operates with an all-volunteer staff. These volunteers often like to joke that they are part of a "budget-free organization." Even if a school is not a member of CUFBA, they can still benefit from their resources. CUFBA offers open-source tools and resources online and free to all. For members, they provide additional access to personalized consulting, and many team members travel to campuses, at cost, to support the development of a campus pantry program. This willingness to provide resources through accessible and open-source methods is one of the key reasons why CUFBA has been so influential in shaping the ways in which colleges and universities design and implement their campus pantry programs.

CUFBA recognizes the uniqueness of each campus, knowing that variables such as student population, location, available resources, potential partnerships off campus, and commitment of campus leaders will impact how a pantry program is developed. At the same time, the CUFBA leadership focuses on a specific model for campus pantry design that efficiently delivers food to students in an accessible manner such that students feel cared for and respected. The key components of this model include having support for the program at the highest possible levels of administration, partnering with a 501(c)(3) nonprofit organization to access food through a local food bank, hosting the pantry in a dedicated space where students feel comfortable, staffing the pantry with persons whose time is dedicated to the program, developing a referral network or additional services to ensure that students' needs are met, collecting and using program data, and only opening a campus pantry program once a sustainability plan is in place. These areas will be discussed now in further detail.

Support from Leadership

The key to success for any campus pantry, particularly at the start, is to have support for the program at the highest levels of leadership possible. The ideal is to have the president of the college or university actively and willing provide resources and utilize their influence to get the program started and sustained. When the president is not available, a vice president or provost can often be a great catalyst for a campus pantry program. What makes this kind of support so critical is that campus leaders are often able to offer what is needed to start a new program or initiative—funding, staff, and space. Space to house a campus pantry program is challenging to obtain on many campuses. Internal politics or scarcity of space often make it impossible for persons who are not in leadership to access a campus planning committee, let alone influence their decisions. Unless the person or persons championing the program already have space available to them, they are likely to have to go to someone more senior to request it. Staffing also often requires approval, either to hire someone new or to structure a current employee's job description to include management of a pantry. Securing funding for staff, as well as things such as position descriptions and the ability to post a new job, is easier when senior leaders are involved. Funding is the most obvious need when starting a new program, and sometimes it can be obtained through grant writing or fundraising without leadership support. However, the best sustainability plan for a campus pantry includes institutionalization of some (or all) of the budget. If that is to be secured, there needs to be buy-in from those who both write and approve budgets. Finally, in a world of tightening higher education budgets it is necessary to have those who make decisions about what programs to keep or cut as supporters of the pantry program. This could include not only the college president but also the board of regents, as well as potentially influential alumni.

There are cases in which campus pantries have been created without leadership support at an institution. The pantry program at OSU was started by students using student fee funding, and space was secured by students through participation in a funding process available to all organizations and units on campus. Even the full-time staff member and student staff who oversaw the pantry functions were funded by the students. There was a need for leaders on campus to approve and oversee the hiring of the staff member, but students were the primary leaders in the hiring process, and the level of leadership needed for this was not the most senior. This example is more an anomaly than it is the norm, and it is much easier to sustain a program when campus leaders are involved. At a minimum, senior leadership cannot be opposed to a pantry program starting on their campus. In all cases where CUFBA provided support to colleges but the president or vice president did not want to have a program on their campus, the program never successfully started.

Partnering with a Nonprofit Organization

Another important recommendation that CUFBA makes is that a campus pantry should develop a relationship with a nonprofit entity that has a 501(c)(3) status. While there are rare cases in which a campus pantry has its own 501(c)(3) designation,[6] most are not allowed to create a nonprofit inside of the institution. A partnership with an off-campus nonprofit fiscal sponsor can make it possible for the program staff or pantry development team to reach out to their local food bank for the purpose of getting food. This can be highly beneficial for the campus pantry, as it allows them to get food to distribute for free or at a fraction of market cost. Even purchases of pantry items in bulk cannot match the affordability of food from a local food bank. Developing such an arrangement requires a few things. First, the college needs to find an appropriate fiscal sponsor that holds a 501(c)(3) nonprofit designation and is willing to share it with the campus pantry. In many cases, the fiscal sponsor also needs to be willing to hold funding for the campus pantry and oversee monetary transactions with the local food bank. This would include receipt of donation or grant dollars, as well as ensuring that any fees associated with getting food from the local food bank are paid. There are many options for the type of nonprofit with which a campus can partner, with common options being another hunger relief agency or the campus foundation.

Partnering with a hunger relief organization not only may provide fiscal sponsorship but also can create opportunities for the campus pantry staff to learn from experts in addressing food insecurity. While those running campus pantries may be well versed in student needs or development theory, they are not always strong on issues like managing inventory, educating clientele, securing foods that may not be available through the local food bank, or networking with other organizations and resources in the community. Hunger relief agencies may also benefit from partnership with a campus pantry. Many serve students and can help connect them with additional resources on campus. Others may have clients interested in going to college who would feel that this is a greater possibility if the staff at the hunger relief agency can provide them with a friendly contact on campus so they can learn how to enroll and know what resources are there for them as they start.

Another way to gain fiscal sponsorship is through a partnering with the campus foundation. This type of partnership comes with some desirable advantages. The two main benefits of this arrangement are easier access to payment processes and a simpler way to raise money. When a pantry utilizes their campus foundation as their nonprofit sponsor, they usually have an account with the foundation to hold and manage their money. Because it is very common for campus offices or organizations to have foundation accounts, there are already proven and predictable processes in place for payment of bills or deposit of new funding. The campus pantry is unlikely to have to create new processes for this type of money management, whereas they may have to with a nonprofit sponsor that has no ties to the college. In many cases the finance managers of smaller nonprofits may be volunteers or work only part-time, making it more challenging to access funding.

The option of partnering with a campus foundation is not without potential issues. One downside could be that spending regulations on money held by the foundation may be more stringent than at a nonprofit off campus—particularly at public institutions. There may be restrictions on the funding that preclude certain types of purchases. Additionally, foundation accounts may have a higher minimum balance than would be required were a nonprofit to hold the pantry's dollars. Another issue could be that the relationship between the college and their foundation is such that any funding spent on student support services, including food, would need to be counted as part of a student's financial aid package. Finally, in some areas the local food banks will not recognize the campus foundation as a nonprofit eligible for partnership because it does not focus on hunger relief. In these cases, colleges have either found off-campus nonprofit sponsors or forgone sponsorship altogether. Regardless of what kind of nonprofit the campus pantry partners with, both parties need to ask a lot of questions, and the relationship should be documented and formalized in a contract or memorandum of understanding.

Some colleges or universities do not have fiscal nonprofit sponsorships. In many cases, a college may not opt for this type of partnership because of the requirements set forth by the local food bank. Because many local food banks receive federal aid in the form of food and funding, they are required to be open to the public. Some campuses do not wish to allow nonstudents to utilize food from their pantry. There could be several reasons for this. In the case of colleges in larger cities like New York or Philadelphia, security is so tight that members of the general public cannot get into campus buildings to access their pantry. In others, funding restrictions do not allow for any food purchased to be provided to persons who are not students. Still other campuses disallow those who are not students to access their pantry because the mission of the pantry is to foster student success, making the provision of food to community members outside of their scope of practice. In these instances, the campus pantry must source its food differently, relying on donations, bulk purchases, or even buying food at market price to stock their shelves. Some campus pantries are very successful at this, and some are not. Those that are not are often unable to provide adequate food for their students. Some even shut down.

Dedicated Space

Having a dedicated space where food is stored and students can access it can be a critical component to the success of a campus pantry. CUFBA has set a broad definition for "dedicated space," noting that this can be as small and simple as a filing cabinet or closet in a dean's office or as elaborate as a fully staffed campus center. What makes a dedicated space so ideal is that students who use the pantry will always know where it is and how to access it. This lets them utilize it more efficiently, as well as share with their peers how to access it. It also cuts down on the time and resources needed for outreach, as fliers, signs, and social media can share a fixed location. In some cases, however, campus pantries are implemented in a disbursed manner or as pop-ups using different locations based on availability. On some campuses, a full-scale pantry is not possible, usually owing to a lack of resources or space. Some pantries adopt a model where food is prepackaged—usually into smaller bags—and placed in a variety of locations on campus. Most of these types of campus pantry programs provide smaller amounts of food, and in many instances the food is lighter—snack foods rather than full meals. If this is a model a college chooses to pursue, CUFBA highly recommends that information on other food resources be included in the bags. The benefit of this model is that food can be stored in even the most inaccessible location and bagged by volunteers all at once and distributed to places that do not require a person present when students pick up the food. Based on what the CUFBA team hears from its members, students deal with issues of stigma and shame, and this model could potentially reduce those feelings. This also means, however, that students do not have access to someone who can answer questions or provide referrals or additional resources. In pop-up-style pantries, the pantry often receives all its food at once and distributes it on the same day. Pop-up pantries make it possible for colleges with limited space to still provide students with food, often making use of classrooms or other spaces that are not in use at the time of distribution. These pantries are usually partnered with a nonprofit sponsor since the program does not have space to receive or store donations. The challenges with the pop-up model include students not always knowing the location of distributions and the pantry program not being able to provide students with food outside of distribution hours.

The final way a campus may host a pantry without having a dedicated space is to invite a mobile pantry to come to campus on a regular basis. Mobile pantry programs are housed inside of vans or large buses and can be driven to distribution locations. They are generally staffed by a local food bank or hunger relief agency, though they can have volunteers serve from the campus. The benefits and drawbacks of the mobile pantry model are similar to those of the pop-up model. Another issue in the mobile pantry model is that college staff are not as actively involved in the program and it is not branded for the college. This can lead to students feeling that the program is not for them and possibly not utilizing it. Staff are not able to identify students who may need additional support because they are not present at distributions.

Appropriate Staffing

CUFBA recommends not only that there be a space designated for a pantry program on campus but also that staff time (preferably paid) be allocated. Staffing a pantry with either a full- or part-time person who is an employee of the college has distinct advantages. The most important is that if the pantry program is under the supervision of a campus employee, the program falls under the insurance of the institution. This is helpful both from a risk management perspective and because many nonprofit sponsors or local food banks require that their pantry partners carry insurance. Staff also provide continuity for a program more so than volunteers or student workers, who often will serve for a few semesters and then move on to some other type of involvement. Even if a staff member only has a percentage of their time dedicated to the pantry program, the program will be stronger. There will be opportunities to grow and improve the program, rather than putting energy into new people or losing knowledge and skills through turnover. Having a staff member at the pantry also allows greater visibility for food insecurity as an issue impacting student success and could have positive impacts on student retention and persistence. Staff forge relationships with students, earning their trust and making it possible to help them access additional resources. Some functional areas where staff have been successful in running campus pantry programs are in dean of students offices, counseling offices, wellness centers, academic affairs offices, and offices of civic engagement. Ideally the person overseeing the pantry program would do so as part of a charge to address poverty among students holistically (as mentioned in several chapters in this book). Running the pantry can be part of their role, as can developing new interventions to address students' basic needs, building resource networks, and performing outreach for the programs offered so that students know how to access them.

By recommending paid staff, CUFBA is not suggesting that there is not a place for students or volunteers at a campus pantry. Many, if not all, pantry programs benefit from either paid student workers or unpaid volunteers. Some do an excellent job of creating development and leadership opportunities for students, placing them in charge of critical components of pantry maintenance such as inventory, ordering, running food drives, and training volunteers. Programs housed in service learning offices often partner with faculty to create cocurricular opportunities for students both to volunteer and to learn about poverty in their community. Student government, clubs and organizations, fraternities and sororities, and even sports teams can play a role in supporting and promoting the campus pantry. At MSU, much of the revenue that keeps the pantry program running is raised by soliciting donations at sporting events. On other campuses, the pantry is the beneficiary of philanthropic endeavors in the Greek community. In many cases, pantry programs have so much support and volunteer interest that they are unable to provide volunteer opportunities for everyone seeking to participate.

Referral Network

As their membership and the number of pantry programs grew, the CUFBA team began to get more and more questions about how campus pantry programs can serve the additional needs of students. CUFBA advises colleges to recognize that the pantry program at a college cannot operate in a vacuum. Instead, it is necessary to develop interconnected networks of resources and services that students can access to meet not only their immediate need for food but other basic needs as well. This can include help with housing, utilities, auto repair, transportation costs, childcare, textbook costs, and longer-term food needs. CUFBA encourages colleges to build relationships with other organizations on and off campus that may be good sources for students as they seek additional assistance. This is where having dedicated staff becomes very helpful. They can go out onto campus and into the community both to learn what is available and to create effective referral pathways to make it easier for students to access additional services. One great example of this is a relationship developed between a campus pantry and a local homeless shelter. When they come across a student experiencing homelessness, the staff at the pantry are trained to do a full intake for the shelter right on campus, making it possible for the student to be admitted to the shelter without having to retell their story to a stranger. The shelter also offers to waive limits on the number of nights students can stay, instead allowing students to remain at the shelter as long as they need while they are still making academic progress toward a credential or degree. When campus pantry programs maintain these types of positive relationships, students can access far more resources than just food.

Data-Driven Approach

Data are critical to the longevity and growth of a campus pantry program. All pantry programs regardless of model, size, space, or staffing should collect as much information as possible on the students they serve, the food (or other items) they distribute, and the services they provide. While the CUFBA team knows that many programs are spread so thinly that they do not have the time or resources to engage in data collection, it is still not considered an optional practice when running a campus pantry. The purpose of this data collection is to help pantry staff make determinations about how to improve and grow the pantry. It is also critical to the long-term sustainability of the pantry, as it provides evidence of the impact of the program. Initially, many pantries measure impact in terms of how many pounds of food they are serving or how many students are receiving support. This is useful information, as it helps demonstrate the need on campus. Combining that information with demographic data on the kinds of students utilizing the pantry may help inform outreach practices, as well as tell the story of the students for whom the program was designed. Many CUFBA members wish to determine a way to track the academic outcomes of students who utilize the pantry, seeking at minimum correlates between pantry usage and persistence and completion rates. This has yet to be done, but the CUFBA team believes that pairing data on academic outcomes with qualitative data from the students in the form of surveys or interviews could provide staff with the confidence that the program is working and justify its existence as part of student success initiatives on campus. It is recommended that staff managing a pantry develop a relationship with either someone in the institutional research office on campus or a faculty member who can support this type of data collection and analysis.

Finally, participating in research such as the #RealCollege Survey, an annual survey measuring food insecurity on college campuses done in partnership with colleges by the Hope Center for College, Community, and Justice, can provide data to demonstrate need for the pantry, as well as make a case for additional services to be developed. Engaging in this kind of data collection and research also contextualizes the need on a specific college or university campus within the national phenomenon of food insecurity among students. This can be very persuasive to skeptics who do not think that food insecurity is a problem on their campus, and it can become a springboard for greater cultural or systemic change beyond the creation of siloed initiatives.

Sustainability Plan   *Hardest*

CUFBA believes that campus pantry programs should have a long-term plan for sustainability, prior to opening. It is more ethical to do nothing than to create a situation that prolongs students' enrollment without the real promise of college completion. While this may seem counterintuitive, it is important to think about the opportunity costs of college enrollment—particularly for low-income students. Each semester that students enroll is time that they may be accruing debt and not working as much in order to be in class. Students sacrifice a great deal to be in school, often sharing with CUFBA members that they are hoping for a better life for themselves and their families. If a campus chooses to step up and support them, they should be prepared to do so throughout the entire time the student is in attendance. This is not to say that if a college cannot open a pantry with 10 (or even 5) years of secured funding, they should not open one. A pantry could have initial funding and combine that with a fundraising plan to pay for it over time to demonstrate their commitment to the sustainability of the program. What is important is that the plan is in place and the pantry has the resources it needs to implement it. Students who utilize campus pantries are vulnerable, and it is important to create a pantry program with that in mind. Developing a program that may really help but is not sustainable could leave students with no choice but to drop out—often with debt.

The most effective way to start a pantry program sustainably is to have all or some of the program funded through the general operating budget of the institution. This demonstrates a commitment from campus leaders who control funding for programs and can remove some of the stressors and challenges of securing donations or grants to cover the costs of the program. The simplest option to institutionalize the program budget is to fund a position to run the pantry and any other poverty alleviation programs that are created around it. This person can start by designing and opening the program and then move on to maintaining its day-to-day functions while engaging in sustainability activities such as collecting and analyzing data to demonstrate the pantry program's impacts and raising money.

Campus Pantry Research

One of the biggest gaps in the national work around campus pantries is the lack of research demonstrating their impacts on student success. At the writing of this book, CUFBA is not aware of any scientifically rigorous studies that have been or are being conducted to measure the efficacy of providing students with food through a campus pantry. The closest is an ongoing experimental study of the Houston Community College (HCC) Food Scholarship Program, where students get groceries from the Houston Food Bank twice per month at farmer's market–style food pantries set up in parking lots adjacent to HCC campuses.[7] Currently, however, there is not strong evidence indicating that campus pantries actually help students stay in college and complete a credential or degree. This is concerning since so many colleges and universities are addressing food insecurity among their students through the creation of a campus pantry. It is important for this research gap to be filled in order to either affirm that campus pantries are a good way to address student food insecurity or engage in a shift of focus to other methods that work better.

One area where research has been conducted on campus pantries is in how they are being implemented. In 2018, CUFBA partnered with the Hope Center for College, Community, and Justice to field a survey of its members, asking them to report on program information such as how long it took to start the program, staffing, space, budget, and types of food being offered. Of the pantries that completed the survey, the majority hosted their program in a dedicated space, and very few had budgets that suggest significant monetary investment in the pantry program.[8] More than half took a year or less to open once the decision was made to start a pantry, and they were started by a broad range of stakeholders, including students, staff, faculty, and community members.[9] More than half serve students exclusively, and over half reported having a nonprofit fiscal sponsor.[10] The biggest challenges that the survey respondents reported were a lack of resources—funds, food, and volunteers being the most common lacking resources.[11] The data released in this report have been well received by CUFBA members, many sharing that they have been using it to press their campus leadership to make changes in their programs or to validate the choices they made in the design of their pantry. CUFBA leadership drew from the results that their recommendations about how to create and run pantry programs have been influential in shaping how the work is being done nationally. For them, it creates an even greater sense of urgency for conducting research on whether pantries have a positive impact on student academic success, well-being, or development.

Conclusion

The future of the organization is now being developed by drawing on CUFBA's most impactful lessons from six years of work in the field: food insecurity among students is a systemic problem requiring systemic solutions, the strength of an organization lies in the relationships between its leaders and its members, and it is only through thoughtful and strategic partnerships that the problem of student hunger will be solved. In 2019, Nate and I stepped down as directors of the organization, with Sonal Chauhan and Brandon Mathews taking on that role. This leadership transition was done with the hope of opening new possibilities for the work through new and innovative leadership.

Innovation is underway to bring CUFBA in better alignment with the needs of the field. With the increase in online resources available for campuses starting programs, as well as their ability to reach out to more and more colleges to learn from, the CUFBA team has observed a drop in the number of requests for direct support. In response to this, the new CUFBA leadership is reevaluating its work and mission to determine next steps for the future. A new website is being designed to address the needs of the field, and in 2018 CUFBA became an official nonprofit with a 501(c)(3) designation, changing from an informal digital community to a formal legal entity. As these changes unfold, the CUFBA team looks forward to reimagining its work and impacts on addressing food insecurity among students.

Addressing food insecurity on college campuses on a national scale is also changing. More and more programs beyond the campus pantry are being conceived and implemented. Many of these are paired with a campus pantry, even having their roots in pantry work prior to being created. While the CUFBA team has gotten fewer and fewer requests to help start a pantry, they have observed an increase in questions about what to do when providing a food box is not enough. When students come to a pantry to get food, they know that the people giving it to them care about them and their well-being. They entrust pantry staff with their stories, which include other issues such as homelessness, lack of transportation, inability to pay for childcare, and other poverty-related challenges. It is becoming increasingly clear that a campus pantry is not adequate to address all the needs of students experiencing food insecurity. Additional services and supports are needed if students are to be served in a manner that addresses their needs fully. Colleges must create interconnected networks to refer students to other services and ensure that they receive them. They must help students gain access to longer-term and more stable sources of food such as the Supplemental Nutrition Assistance Program, create programs that offer food subsidies or scholarships, or more broadly address the full price of college attendance so that students have the funds to pay for food. Through assisting colleges as they start campus pantries, CUBFA has helped to uncover a crucial truth about food insecurity on college campuses: it takes a multifaceted approach to address this issue and all of the symptoms of poverty students are dealing with while pursuing college education.

CUFBA believes that there is a role for the campus pantry within this multifaceted approach. Pantries serve to get people in the door. They draw students in, providing them today with the food they needed yesterday, and allowing them to share with college staff what they are going to need tomorrow. Pantries also bring colleges into the movement, engaging them in the important work of addressing poverty on their campuses and opening the door for them to do more than hand out boxes of food. It cannot be *the* solution, but it is a gateway into one—a gateway more and more campuses are walking through each year, seeking to secure success for their students.

Notes

1. The oldest known campus pantries started in the early 1990s. Sara Goldrick-Rab, Clare Cady, and Vanessa Coca, *Campus Food Pantries: Insights from a National Survey* (Philadelphia: Hope Center for College, Community, and Justice, 2018), https://hope4college.com/wp-content/uploads/2018/09/2018-CUFBA-Report-web-2.pdf.

2. M. Pia Chaparro et al., "Food Insecurity Prevalence among College Students at the University of Hawai'i at Manōa," *Public Health Nutrition* 12, no. 11 (2009): 2097–103; Roger Hughes et al., "Student Food Insecurity: The Skeleton in the University Closet," *Nutrition and Dietetics* 68, no. 1 (2011): 27–32.

3. "Resources," College and University Food Bank Alliance, https://www.cufba.org.

4. James Dubick, Brandon Mathews, and Clare Cady, *Hunger on Campus: The Challenge of Food Insecurity and College Students* (Boston: National Student Campaign Against Hunger and Homelessness, 2016), https://studentsagainsthunger.org/hunger-on-campus/.

5. Sara Goldrick-Rab, Katharine M. Broton, and Daniel Eisenberg, *Hungry to Learn: Addressing Food and Housing Insecurity among Undergraduates* (Madison: Wisconsin HOPE Lab, 2015), https://hope4college.com/wp-content/uploads/2018/09/Wisconsin_HOPE_Lab_Hungry_To_Learn.pdf.

6. "About the Food Bank," MSU Student Food Bank, http://foodbank.msu.edu/about/index.html.

7. Sara Goldrick-Rab, Katharine M. Broton, and Daphne C. Hernandez, *Addressing Basic Needs Security in Higher Education: An Introduction to Three Evaluations of Supports for Food and Housing at Community Colleges* (Madison: Wisconsin HOPE Lab, 2017), https://hope4college.com/wp-content/uploads/2018/09/Addressing-Basic-Needs-Security-in-Higher-Education.pdf.

8. Sara Goldrick-Rab, Clare Cady, and Vanessa Coca, *Campus Food Pantries: Insights from a National Survey* (Philadelphia: Hope Center for College, Community, and Justice, 2018), https://hope4college.com/wp-content/uploads/2018/09/2018-CUFBA-Report-web-2.pdf.

9. Goldrick-Rab, Cady, and Coca, *Campus Food Pantries*, 6.

10. Goldrick-Rab, Cady, and Coca, *Campus Food Pantries*, 7.

11. Goldrick-Rab, Cady, and Coca, *Campus Food Pantries*, 1.

[3]

The American Federation of Teachers Local 212 / MATC FAST (Faculty and Students Together) Fund

MICHAEL ROSEN

Editors' Prologue. Experiences of food insecurity and hunger rarely occur in isolation. Instead, students struggling to make ends meet constantly juggle how they will pay for tuition, fees, books and supplies, housing, food, transportation, childcare, and other basic necessities. This chapter explains how a faculty-led approach to emergency grant aid helps students get enough to eat by helping them afford housing, food, and other expenses that can derail students' academic success if not met in a timely manner. Furthermore, it illustrates the systemic nature of basic needs insecurity by explaining the socioeconomic, historical, and political context of a major American city. Though the chapter focuses on a community college in Milwaukee, Wisconsin, we believe that the demonstrated mechanisms and processes are widespread, providing essential insights for anyone seeking to better understand and serve today's undergraduates.

About the Author. Michael Rosen is the founder and director of the Local 212/MATC Believe in Students FAST Fund. He retired in May 2016 from the Milwaukee Area Technical College, where he taught economics for 29 years. For 17 years he served as the president of the faculty union, the American Federation of Teachers Local 212. He has a PhD in urban studies from the University of Wisconsin–Milwaukee.

Rosalind, a student with a 3.5 grade point average (GPA), was one semester away from completing her nursing degree at Milwaukee Area Technical College (MATC) when she became homeless. Her personal relationship had been rocky. But after an incident when her boyfriend kicked and punched her, she left. As Rosalind explained, "I learned in class that women who are abused don't try to move out until they've been hit seven times. When my fiancé's verbal abuse turned physical, I decided once was enough. I left that night while he was asleep with the few possessions I could take with me."[1]

With no place to turn, her car and a local gas station became her home. After a few days, she moved in with her sister's family, sleeping on the floor because the couch and beds were occupied. But that did not last: the landlord evicted the entire family for violating their lease, which limited the number of people residing in the apartment.

Rosalind, a full-pay student like many in community colleges, had exhausted her federal financial aid eligibility because of the notorious 150 percent rule that denies students financial aid once they have completed 150 percent of the credits needed to graduate from their program, regardless of the circumstances.[2] This is not an uncommon experience among low-income, first-generation students who are forced to navigate the world of higher education with no mentor while juggling work, school, and family responsibilities.

After graduating from a northern Wisconsin high school, Rosalind enrolled in the University of Wisconsin–Whitewater. She completed three years toward a biomedical degree. Her goal was to become a veterinarian. However, after working at a hospital, she realized that people were her real passion. She transferred to Gateway Technical College, one of sixteen colleges in the Wisconsin Technical College System, where she completed her prerequisites. But Gateway had a multiyear waiting list for its nursing program. So Rosalind applied to MATC's nursing program and was accepted.

While a Pell Grant and Wisconsin Covenant Scholars Grant helped her pay for her first few years at Whitewater, they were not enough to cover her tuition, books, and living expenses. She worked and took out loans to cover what financial aid did not. As a result, Rosalind, one semester short of earning her nursing degree, found herself homeless with a student debt of nearly $40,000 despite working full-time as a certified nursing assistant/health unit coordinator.

After being evicted from her sister's place, Rosalind found a modest apartment in the suburban community of her required nursing clinical placement. She earned enough to cover the rent but did not have funds for the security deposit. She applied for a small emergency grant from MATC's Dreamkeepers program, which is designed to provide financial support to students for one-time, unexpected events that impede their ability to stay in school. However, the program only assists students who are current Pell Grant recipients.[3] Since Rosalind had exhausted her financial aid eligibility and no longer received a Pell Grant, MATC's Dreamkeepers program denied her request for emergency financial assistance. That is when she contacted the American Federation of Teachers (AFT) Local 212/MATC Believe in Students FAST (Faculty and Students Together) Fund, a faculty union–initiated, emergency resource for MATC students.

The FAST Fund contacted her nursing instructor, whom Rosalind had listed as her faculty reference—the same faculty member who had urged Rosalind to contact the FAST Fund. Rosalind received a glowing recommendation from the instructor. The FAST Fund wrote a check to the landlord covering the security deposit. Rosalind now had a roof over her head near her fall clinical placement. She graduated as a registered nurse in December 2018, passed her state boards the following month, and is now employed as a nurse making $30 an hour.

Rosalind's experience is not atypical. Eviction, homelessness, and food insecurity are major problems experienced by MATC students. In response to financial crises like these, the AFT Local 212/MATC Believe in Students FAST Fund was launched in September 2016.

Milwaukee: Context for the AFT Local 212 / MATC Believe in Students FAST Fund

Milwaukee was selected as one of the nation's first FAST Fund sites because it is one of the nation's poorest cities.[4] The former manufacturing hub was once a stable, blue-collar, middle-class city known as the nation's biggest small town. But Milwaukee has been devastated by deindustrialization and deunionization, hemorrhaging family-supporting jobs and impoverishing residential neighborhoods. Between 1979 and 1983, Milwaukee lost more manufacturing jobs, 56,000, than it lost during the Great Depression.[5]

Major unionized employers like Allis Chalmers, A. O. Smith, Continental Can, and American Motors that once employed tens of thousands of workers have closed their doors. Others that remain, such as Master Lock, Briggs and Stratton, Allen Bradley, Ember Meatpacking, and Harley Davidson, have significantly reduced employment.[6] Commercial districts that thrived adjacent to these mammoth factories, as well as the bars, restaurants, credit unions, sporting goods stores, and auto repair shops that served their blue-collar, middle-class workers, collapsed as employment and discretionary income plummeted.

According to Marc Levine, director of the University of Wisconsin–Milwaukee Center for Economic Development, "The loss of manufacturing employment, the historical backbone of family-supporting jobs and economic prosperity in Milwaukee, has been relentless and substantial since the 1970s. After peaking in 1963, manufacturing employment has declined by over 77 percent in the city of Milwaukee. In 1970, manufacturing employment represented almost 36 percent of the city's job base; today, less than 10 percent of the city's jobs are in manufacturing. In the 1960s, almost 60 percent of metro Milwaukee's industrial jobs were located in the city; today, less than 19 percent of regional manufacturing takes place in the city of Milwaukee."[7]

Deindustrialization has been accompanied by a precipitous decline in union jobs. While estimates vary, some researchers estimate that 30–40 percent of the rise in inequality in the past 30 years is because of the decline of unions. As Schmitt and Jones conclude,

> The decline in the economy's ability to create good jobs is related to deterioration in the bargaining power of workers, especially those at the middle and bottom of the pay scale. The restructuring of the U.S. labor market—including the decline in the inflation-adjusted value of the minimum wage, the fall in unionization, deregulation, pro-corporate trade agreements, a dysfunctional immigration system, and macroeconomic policy that has with few exceptions kept unemployment well above the full employment level—has substantially reduced the bargaining power of U.S. workers, effectively pulling the bottom out of the labor market and increasing the share of bad jobs in the economy.[8]

During the 1950s and 1960s, when manufacturing was ascendant, 35–40 percent of Milwaukee's labor force was unionized. By 1986, that percentage had fallen to slightly less than 26 percent. Today only 11 percent of metro Milwaukee workers are covered by union contracts, and only 5 percent of private sector workers are covered. As Levine notes, "Even in sectors that were formerly union strongholds, such as manufacturing, the unionization rate has precipitously fallen, which helps explain why real wages fell for production workers in metro Milwaukee between 2000–2012 by 6.4 percent."[9] Those who found work in the service sector are paid significantly less. Princeton University professor Matthew Desmond explains, "Machinists in the old Allis Chalmers plant earned $11.60 an hour; clerks in the shopping center that replaced much of that plant in 1987 earned $5.23."[10] From 1979 to 2010, as Milwaukee experienced deindustrialization and deunionization, household incomes dropped 12 percent when adjusted for inflation. During the decade between 1981 and 1991, the number of high-poverty census tracks in Milwaukee tripled, more than any other city in the country.[11]

The impact on Milwaukee's black community, home to roughly 30 percent of MATC's students, has been nothing short of a "silent depression," as black household incomes dropped a startling 28.9 percent between 1979 and 2010.[12] In 1970, prior to the collapse of the unionized manufacturing sector, the city's black family median income was 19 percent higher than the national median. By 2000, even before the Great Recession, Milwaukee's median black family income was 23 percent lower than the national median—a swing of 42 percentage points. Milwaukee's black poverty in 1970 was 22 percent lower than the national black poverty rate. By 2000, Milwaukee's black poverty rate was 34 percent higher than the national rate, the highest in the nation's twenty largest cities.[13]

Milwaukee is also one of the nation's most hypersegregated communities. The standard measure of segregation used by sociologists is the "index of dissimilarity." It represents the share of a group's population that would have to move for each neighborhood to have the same share of that group in the city overall. According to Dr. Levine,

> A measure of 60 is considered "high" segregation; 80 is considered "extreme" segregation. By 1970, the black-white index of dissimilarity in Milwaukee was 90.5, and it has never dipped below 80 since. By 1980, using five different indicators of segregation (dissimilarity, isolation, clustering, centralization, and concentration), researchers identified Milwaukee as one of the nation's most *hypersegregated* large metropolitan areas, ranking in the top five on *each* of these indicators. . . . Even as major metro areas across the U.S. have modestly desegregated since the 1980s, Milwaukee's rate of black-white segregation has barely budged. Not only has Milwaukee persistently ranked among the nation's most racially segregated metropolitan areas since 1970, but in contrast to many of the country's historically most segregated regions, the residential segregation of African Americans has barely diminished in Milwaukee over the past thirty years.[14]

Despite the city's increased poverty and segregation, rents remain very high. In areas where minorities make up at least 25 percent of the population, the median rent is $892. As a result, evictions are a common occurrence in the high-poverty African American neighborhoods. In *Evicted: Poverty and Profit in an American City*, Matthew Desmond documents that "women from black neighborhoods made up 9 percent of Milwaukee's population and 30 percent of its evicted tenants."[15] He writes, "between 2009 and 2011 more than 1 in 8 Milwaukee renters experienced a forced move."[16]

More than half of MATC's students come from these hypersegregated and impoverished neighborhoods. Forty percent are the first in their families to attend college. Further, 61 percent of MATC students rely on federal financial aid to help pay for their college education.[17]

If we want to ensure that our students succeed, we need to design programs and support services that address the reality of their lives. This requires more than good intentions. The challenges our students face and the choices they make are informed by their history and the socioeconomic conditions they have experienced. Deindustrialization, deunionization, and segregation created the neighborhoods our students live in, the labor markets they work in, the careers they choose, and the programs they select when they enroll in college in pursuit of stable employment and a successful career. While a postsecondary credential was not always necessary for their parents or grandparents to earn a living wage, this is no longer true for most young adults. Although these patterns of racial and economic inequality are particularly pronounced in Milwaukee, they are found in virtually every major American city. The loss of manufacturing jobs, the decline in union membership and clout, the decline in real wages, and the growth of the service sector are impacting higher education in the United States and reshaping labor markets.

Establishing and Funding the AFT Local 212 / MATC Believe in Students FAST Fund

The AFT Local 212 / MATC FAST Fund is student centered, faculty led, and housed in the local union office on campus. It began with a

$5,000 grant from Believe in Students Inc.—a nonprofit organization founded by Dr. Sara Goldrick-Rab in order to establish and support FAST Funds across the nation.[18] Dr. Goldrick-Rab is a professor of higher education policy and sociology at Temple University and a leading expert on financial aid. She created the FAST Fund to "help make students' immediate survival possible while others work to create the systemic change to solve the root causes of this problem."[19] Like FAST Funds at other colleges, the AFT Local 212/MATC FAST Fund is a nonprofit affiliate of Believe in Students Inc.

Dr. Goldrick-Rab and University of Wisconsin HOPE Lab scholars had interviewed MATC students during the summer and fall of 2016 for their study of college student food insecurity and homelessness. It was clear from her research and these interviews at Wisconsin's only majority-minority college that major economic challenges, including housing and food insecurity, unreliable transportation, other costs associated with attending college, and the 150 percent rule covering eligibility for federal financial aid, are significant obstacles for MATC students.[20]

Pell Grants and other forms of financial aid do not cover the real cost of college attendance for MATC's primarily low-income students, the majority of whom are residents of Milwaukee.[21] Despite working long hours at mainly low-paying jobs, when a crisis such as illness, a reduction in work hours, a death in the family, or car trouble hits, students struggle to attend classes, complete assignments, and even remain enrolled. Students cannot focus on their studies when they do not know where their next meal is coming from. The FAST Fund was organized to provide rapid, hassle-free support to students experiencing financial emergencies.

Including the $5,000 start-up grant from Believe in Students Inc., the FAST Fund raised $119,180 between 2016 and April 2019. During its first year, AFT Local 212 raised $2,500 from concerned faculty and retirees at a reception featuring Dr. Goldrick-Rab following the publication of her book *Paying the Price: College Costs,*

Financial Aid, and the Betrayal of the American Dream. MATC's faculty and retirees have been the FAST Fund's most consistent source of revenue. Their contributions have been complemented by support from the broader community.

MATC's faculty know that many of their students survive on the nation's economic margins, where a loss in work hours, a delayed financial aid check, the loss of a childcare provider, an eviction, or a layoff can make regular attendance and completion of homework assignments very difficult. MATC's faculty members experience this reality in their students' attendance and performance. When students fall asleep in class, it is often because they worked all night or until early hours in the morning. Assignments may be late or incomplete because students do not have internet service at home, their kids got sick, or students are too exhausted to study after working long hours at one, two, or even three jobs. As a result, MATC's faculty and retirees have been extraordinarily supportive of the FAST Fund, a living refutation of the myth that teachers and their unions are narrow and selfish.

The FAST Fund raised an additional $47,000 for the 2017–18 academic year. In the spring of 2017, I retired after 29 years on the MATC faculty, the last 17 as the president of AFT Local 212. I asked colleagues to contribute to the FAST Fund in lieu of gifts. Prior to the retirement dinner held in my honor, faculty, retirees, and friends had contributed $6,000. At the dinner an anonymous donor matched that, and we collected pledges of an additional $4,000. In July 2017, AFT Local 212 issued a press release about the FAST Fund and its successful fundraising. The story was picked up by the state's major newspaper, the *Milwaukee Journal Sentinel*.[22] That generated another $4,000 from a variety of people unaffiliated with MATC or AFT Local 212 who empathized with MATC's students.

The FAST Fund has continued to raise funds over the years. During MATC's 2017–18 annual Giving Campaign, the fund received almost $1,900 in contributions from faculty members who wrote in the nonprofit's name. The fund is working to be listed as an official recipient. The fund has also presented at MATC retiree meetings and sent emails and letters to retirees and active members explaining its work and soliciting funds.

In December 2017, Dr. Goldrick-Rab won the University of Louisville Grawemeyer Award in Education for her 2016 book, *Paying the Price: College Costs, Financial Aid, and the Betrayal of the American Dream*, and for her research and advocacy on behalf of low-income students. Dr. Goldrick-Rab offered to match any new contributions to FAST Funds on a three-to-one basis until her $100,000 Grawemeyer prize was exhausted.[23] The AFT Local 212 FAST Fund immediately sent out a solicitation explaining the matching grant. That campaign raised nearly $30,000, including Goldrick-Rab's match.

More recently, the FAST Fund raised almost $6,500 at a morning benefit concert at a local coffee shop. The fund has also reached out to local foundations, and last year it was awarded a $5,000 grant from the Kohl Foundation. In February 2019, the FAST Fund held its first annual gala and silent auction. The gala sold out. The auction, which was supported by the Green Bay Packers, the Milwaukee Bucks, and many local restaurants and businesses, including several of which are owned by MATC graduates, raised $25,500. The FAST Fund continues to pursue a variety of fundraising strategies in order to help MATC students.

Helping Students

In its first year, 2016–17, the FAST Fund spent its entire $7,500 budget to assist 23 students. The most frequent need (9 out of 23 students, or 39%) was preventing evictions and/or securing housing for homeless students. Fifteen of the 23 were female students. The fund's experience confirmed the findings of Princeton University professor Mathew Desmond, who wrote about Milwaukee in *Evicted: Poverty and Profit in an American City*, "If incarceration had come to define the lives of men from impoverished black neighborhoods [in Milwaukee], eviction was shaping the lives of women. Poor black men were locked up. Poor black women were locked out."[24] Nine additional students were helped with various other "costs of attendance" such as food, books, tools, and fees for health science students' testing and equipment. These fees are often unadvertised and unexpected, but they are significant enough to prevent students from pursuing their education.

In 2017–18, the FAST Fund helped more than 100 students. Addressing housing insecurity by assisting students in either avoiding eviction or securing housing was the single largest area of need, accounting for 43 of the cases. Other issues the fund helped address were the cost of college, 20; auto assistance, 18; and tuition assistance, 12. Tuition support was provided to several students who were limited by the 150 percent rule or were full-pay Deferred Action for Childhood Arrivals (DACA) students. The FAST Fund only helped three food-insecure students. That should not be interpreted to mean that MATC students do not experience food insecurity. Food is often the first thing that students sacrifice. Students report routinely skipping meals to pay for books or to pay their rent. Jennifer, a student in the MATC Adult Promise program, reflected on her experience: "I have had to make tough decisions. I've skipped lots of meals trying to juggle things. You want to cry you get so hungry, but you have no choice. You want to ask for help, but you feel ashamed to ask. So you go hungry and just try to make it."[25]

The FAST Fund frequently refers food-insecure students to the college food pantry, community food pantries and kitchens, and the Dreamkeepers emergency grant program. The Hunger Task Force, a Milwaukee-area anti-hunger organization, has a staff person assigned to the college, and Saint Ben's, a community-based meal site for the homeless and working poor run by the Capuchin Franciscan ministry, is just two blocks from MATC's downtown campus. Nonetheless, the FAST Fund experienced a large increase in demand by food-insecure students in 2018–19 because Dreamkeepers—MATC's emergency grant aid program—no longer provides students with food. As a result, food insecurity has become the second-largest area of expenditure for the FAST Fund, second only to housing insecurity.

Utility requests are handled similarly. Students who seek utility assistance are encouraged to apply to the Wisconsin Energy Assistance program, for example. Referrals for food, utilities, and other basic needs are made to maximize the FAST Funds' resources for other areas of need that are not addressed by community agencies. Collaboration with community resources provides the fund with the flexibility it needs to fill gaps in the existing student support system.

In 2017–18, the FAST Fund helped students from every MATC school and from the following programs: accounting, automotive technology, aviation, biotechnology, business management, chemical technician, culinary arts, culinary management, dental technician, diesel and powertrain servicing, dietetic technician, early childhood education, electricity, human services, heating ventilation and air conditioning, internet technology networking, liberal arts, legal administration professional, marketing management, masonry, nursing, nursing assistant, paralegal, police science, precollege and business, radiography, real estate, and television and video production.

Coordination with MATC Dreamkeepers Emergency Grant Program

As noted above, the FAST Fund works closely with MATC and community-based programs in order to stretch limited resources and serve students. Since its inception, the FAST Fund has worked to coordinate with MATC's significantly richer emergency funds, and a strong collaborative relationship has developed.

The MATC Dreamkeepers funds are governed by more stringent rules, established by external funders, than the FAST Fund. These include an application process many students find difficult, a one-time maximum distribution of $500, documentation of need, and a minimum turnaround of 48 hours, but often taking much longer. To qualify for a Dreamkeepers emergency grant, a student must be receiving a Pell Grant, have an MATC cumulative GPA of at least 2.0, and be experiencing a one-time emergency. While this program is an important resource for some MATC students, these stringent rules are problematic. For instance, DACA students, students who have maximized their financial aid eligibility, and new and transfer students are immediately disqualified. Although MATC does not have data on the number of students at the 150 percent maximum rule, it appears to be a serious impediment to many MATC students. For example, 17 of 54 (31%) students the FAST Fund served during the Spring 2018 semester were paying tuition out of pocket because they had reached the 150 percent maximum credit rule.

Dreamkeepers is designed for a single emergency such as a stolen computer, an unexpected loss of income, or a car repair. But poverty, particularly extreme poverty, is not a one-time occurrence. As Marcella Bombardieri notes, "Many students lurch from crisis to crisis, semester to semester. That's part of why community college graduation rates are so low."[26]

The FAST Fund, on the other hand, is much more flexible. It is designed to respond to emergencies more rapidly than Dreamkeepers and with a less complex application process. During the FAST Fund's first year of operation, it had no application process at all. The following year, as the number of applicants grew and to keep better records, it established a simple one-page online application. Students are asked basic identification information (name, contact information, and school ID), to explain and document their need, and to provide a faculty reference.

When the FAST Fund reviews students' applications, we consider whether the Dreamkeepers emergency grant program may be a better fit for their needs. If the student is receiving federal financial aid, their emergency is not immediate, and they have not already contacted Dreamkeepers, then the FAST Fund asks them to apply to Dreamkeepers first. The FAST Fund will frequently follow up on the Dreamkeepers application to ensure that it has all the necessary documentation and to help expedite the student request.

If a student is denied by Dreamkeepers, then they are often referred to the FAST Fund, and we will attempt to address their needs. For instance, Priscilla had all of her books and a laptop stolen. She was ineligible for a Dreamkeepers grant because she was a first-semester student and did not have an MATC cumulative GPA of at least 2.0, a Dreamkeepers' requirement. The FAST Fund stepped in to help her. As she explained in an email, "During the fall semester I was in a really, really tough situation because all my books and resources were stolen. I contacted MATC's Dreamkeepers about my situation. Dreamkeepers referred me to the FAST Fund. Thanks to the FAST Fund I recovered my resources. The FAST Fund helped me immensely. I did not fall behind in school because the FAST Fund supported me. . . . Thank you FAST Fund for helping me pass my fall semester of college."[27]

The goal in coordinating with Dreamkeepers and other MATC funds is to provide MATC students with the maximum support possible from all sources. Frequently Dreamkeepers will contact the FAST Fund, asking whether it can co-fund a student. For example, Dreamkeepers recently allocated $500 toward a $980 car repair. The FAST Fund provided the additional $480. Both programs share the goal of helping students overcome financial challenges so they are able to remain focused on their academic work. The FAST Fund's strength lies in the ability to provide rapid assistance with minimal bureaucracy and increased flexibility.

More than Emergency Aid: Advocacy and Leverage of Additional Resources

In addition to providing emergency assistance, the FAST Fund also advocates for students who are not acquainted with MATC and community emergency programs, or who have trouble applying for them. In 2017–18, the FAST Fund leveraged more than $13,000 for MATC students, and it surpassed that number in 2018–19. Since the scope of this advocacy and leverage work is far-reaching, I include several examples to provide the reader with a sense of the work completed by the FAST Fund.

In its first year, the FAST Fund helped an undocumented student, who had been suspended because he owed the college money for the previous semester, secure a $1,200 unused Latino scholarship; helped a Hmong student at the 150 percent credit limit secure a $1,380 tuition grant from the college's completion fund; and even got the college to expedite a Dreamkeepers payment for a student who was an Uber driver when her car was impounded. The FAST Fund secured this student support because it knew that these funds existed and knew whom to call.

In 2017–18, a single, working mother with a 3.8 GPA studying chemical technology was denied Dreamkeepers support because she had exhausted her federal financial aid eligibility. She was in danger of dropping out because she could not afford the tuition. The FAST Fund contacted the MATC Foundation to determine whether she would qualify for a Completion Fund grant, a little-known and little-publicized fund. She did not. But the foundation identified an unused chemical technology scholarship and awarded her $1,000 toward her tuition, allowing her to remain enrolled.

In another case, Dreamkeepers denied a Native American student's request for assistance because she did not have an MATC cumulative GPA of at least 2.0. Jessica was a 3.8 GPA transfer student from Waukesha County Technical College (WCTC) in a partnership program. A single mom, she had completed her prerequisites at WCTC and was enrolled in her clinical, an onsite hospital placement where students work directly with patients under the supervision of faculty. The FAST Fund called the MATC Foundation on the student's behalf and explained her circumstances. Once the MATC staff realized that the student was in a collaborative program, they provided her with the requested emergency funding. Jessica wrote the FAST Fund, "This semester is off to another good start.

For me the fast fund was a huge relief. Your financial help allowed me to focus on my studies rather than my financial situation. If it was not for this fast fund I would have had to drop classes and return to work so I could get caught up financially. This is a great program that was fast and convenient. Thank you so much for your help."[28]

In the fall of 2018, MATC launched the MATC Promise for Adults, a free-tuition, last-dollar program for adults aged 24 years or older who have earned at least six college credits and have been out of school for a minimum of two years.[29] According to MATC president Vicki Martin, 22 percent of all Milwaukee County residents have started but not completed a college degree.[30] As soon as the semester began, Adult Promise students began contacting the FAST Fund because the program did not cover the cost of books and they could not afford them. Employees of the MATC bookstore also contacted the FAST Fund about this problem. AFT Local 212 president Lisa Conley emailed the college president, urging the college administration to address this problem. Dr. Martin committed to providing these students with books. As a result, nine students who were on the verge of dropping out obtained books and remained enrolled. As Mareza, one of the Adult Promise students, wrote,

> Because of your generosity and support I will be able to attend my classes. . . . Thank you so much for purchasing my required text books for the classes I am enrolled for in the 2018 fall semester. In such a short amount of time I was awarded entry into a program leaving me little time to financially prepare for the cost of books. Not only did you greatly impact my decision to continue this semester you also went above and beyond to assure I had text books for my remaining classes as well. In a matter of hours you made it possible for me to continue in the nursing program! Thank you for your dedication and work in the community! You are truly a hero!!![31]

The FAST Fund also promotes MATC scholarships and helps students apply for them. When the college announced that it had secured $10,000 for DACA student summer scholarships, the FAST Fund contacted DACA students it had assisted in the past and other DACA students AFT Local 212 had worked with politically. The fund helped four students apply successfully for these scholarships. As one of the students, Josue, recalled, "The scholarships were a gift from God which I shared with the other DACA students. It's very tough working full-time, having to pay for all of my classes, and trying to keep up with my studies. The FAST Fund helped me get through some tough times."[32]

The FAST Fund has also been creative in utilizing campus programs. For instance, the fund has collaborated with the auto technology program to repair student automobiles. It is a win-win situation because the program needs cars to work on to provide its students with hands-on experience. When a student with a car repair applies to the fund, it calls the auto program instructors to determine whether they can use the car in their instruction. If they can, the program will complete the repair at a significantly reduced cost to the FAST Fund. Similarly, MATC IT staff members were able to save students significant dollars by fixing their computers.

The FAST Fund has also developed relations with other community resources. In addition to helping students apply for emergency energy assistance, the fund has helped several students get new glasses through LensCrafters's OneSight program. This is a program that provides free eye exams and glasses if needed. The only requirement is a referral from a nonprofit organization, public school, or accredited college. When this relationship was first established, the LensCrafters program was run by an MATC graduate, although this is no longer the case. In addition, the FAST Fund has established working relations with local social service and religious organizations, as well as Legal Action's Eviction Project, that provide services useful to students.

Some students who contact the FAST Fund need more than simple financial assistance. However, the faculty members who run the FAST Fund are not social workers or counselors. In such cases, the fund refers students to MATC's counselors so that they can help devise a plan for the students. For example, a working student devoted her entire check to securing stable housing. She then—in desperation—went to the local casino, hoping "that God would help her." She lost her last $200. This was not the first time she had lost money hoping to hit it big. As a condition of support, the FAST Fund required the student to make an appointment and meet with an MATC counselor. They developed a plan that included having the student voluntarily barred from the casino. Once that was accomplished, the FAST Fund provided the student with the requested assistance. Later, the student thanked the FAST Fund for its compassion and assistance.

In short, the FAST Fund provides much more than emergency aid. It has become a hub for students and their advocates. By coordinating with Dreamkeepers, the Wisconsin Emergency Energy program, LensCrafters's OneSight, Saint Ben's, Repairers of the Breach, Community Advocates, academic programs that provide useful services, and other community resources, it helps students exhaust available resources before drawing on FAST Fund dollars. This is a key strategy that maximizes flexibility and allows the FAST Fund to fill the gaps in areas that other resources will not cover.

Faculty Involvement

MATC is a large institution with four campuses and approximately 40,000 students. Like all large institutions, it is often difficult for students to identify and access the resources they need, particularly when they are in crisis. Faculty are the college employees with whom students have the most direct and consistent contact. They are the employees to whom students feel most connected. Students and instructors bond through the course of a semester or even several semesters. This is reflected in student surveys that routinely rank faculty as the college's most valued resource.[33] Because of this consistent and close relationship, faculty members are frequently the first to notice when a student is in crisis. And conversely, students are often most comfortable confiding in their instructors with whom they have bonded. This relationship between students and faculty is central to the FAST Fund's operation and success and why it is important to establish faculty-led emergency funds.

The FAST Fund is faculty led and relies on their support and involvement. Prior to the beginning of the Fall 2017 semester, Dr. Goldrick-Rab encouraged the FAST Fund to help its faculty include in their syllabi a statement encouraging students experiencing economic crisis to talk to their instructor about it so the faculty could connect those students to the FAST Fund. AFT Local 212's president, Dr. Lisa Conley, modified Goldrick-Rab's draft and sent it to all of MATC's faculty, encouraging them to include it in their syllabi. The statement read, *"Housing, Food or Other Insecurity?* If you are having difficulty affording or accessing sufficient food to eat every day, or if you lack a safe and stable place to live, and believe this may affect your performance in this course, I urge you to contact an MATC counselor, the director of Local 212's FAST Fund at 414-467-8908 or MATC's Dreamkeepers emergency fund program at 414-297-7876 for support. Furthermore, please notify me if you are comfortable in doing so. I may be able to provide additional resource information or assistance as appropriate and available."

The inclusion of this paragraph was important for two reasons. It was a clear message to students that their instructors were concerned about their physical and psychological well-being as well as their academic performance and that they understood that these were linked. Several faculty members reported that students confided in them at least in part because they had included the housing and food insecurity statement in their syllabus. In addition, several FAST Fund applicants report that they first learned about the FAST Fund and how to contact it from their syllabus.

Faculty also play a critical role in determining whether a student is eligible for a FAST Fund emergency grant. A faculty reference is required for all applicants. This reference, documentation of need, and an interview with the FAST Fund director are the fund's principal accountability measures.

The faculty reference serves three reinforcing purposes. First, it provides the fund and its donors assurance that the student, despite their challenging circumstances, is committed to pursuing their education and worthy of FAST Fund support. Second, it provides the faculty member important information about nonacademic factors that may be affecting the student's performance. In some cases, faculty members are aware of their students' plight. Many students call the FAST Fund based on instructors' recommendations. But sometimes instructors are not aware. In those cases where the student has not shared their circumstances with their instructors, the FAST Fund's reference call alerts the faculty to nonacademic challenges that may be affecting the student's academic work. Finally, the faculty reference is an effective tool for building support among the faculty for the FAST Fund. Faculty appreciate that the FAST Fund seeks out and relies on their evaluation in making its awards and that it is helping their students succeed and their program maintain enrollment.

The AFT Local 212/MATC FAST Fund is run by AFT Local 212—the MATC faculty union—out of their local union office on campus. Not only does this make the FAST Fund easily accessible to students, but it also provides legitimacy among faculty and staff because AFT Local 212 has represented MATC faculty since 1930.

Faculty-led emergency funds like the FAST Fund are valuable faculty union projects. Housing the FAST Fund within a union, particularly if the (AFT) Local has a history on campus, creates institutional accountability and legitimacy. It also provides the fund with a mechanism for identifying and reaching out to students in need. The AFT Local 212/MATC FAST Fund experience is that the FAST Fund activity is embraced by faculty and retirees who want their union to promote student success and collaboration with community organizations. They have also been the main donor base, consistently contributing to the FAST Fund, which has allowed it to increase the scale of its activity from year one to year two by 361 percent.

The FAST Fund's main purpose is to help students overcome financial crises, remain enrolled, and succeed. But if it is successful, it will help build the local union among members and potential members, a valuable secondary objective in light of the US Supreme Court's *Janus* decision and efforts by right-wing organizations to weaken unions.[34] The Temple Association of University Professionals, the union representing all faculty, professional librarians, and academic professionals, for example, also started a FAST Fund in 2018. Several other AFT Local affiliates, with the help of a challenge grant from Believe in Students Inc., have launched FAST Funds in recent years.[35] Faculty unions are excellent homes for faculty-led emergency aid programs. If the local union model is not applicable, emergency fund projects could be run through faculty senates or be organized as stand-alone entities.

Systemic and Institutional Issues

The FAST Fund is admittedly a Band-Aid. It cannot solve the deeply rooted problems of poverty, inequality, and economic insecurity, which are fundamental characteristics of the United States' economy and labor market. The AFT Local 212 / MATC FAST Fund does what it can with limited resources to assist individual students. But in the long run, the problems of the poor, the number of unemployed and underemployed, poverty, and inequality will continue to grow in Wisconsin and across the nation because they are systemic.[36] Wisconsin has not been unique in aggressively pursuing an economic development strategy based on low wages, reduced taxes and regulations, and privatization rather than investment in higher education.[37] This low-road approach has undermined the ability of low- and moderate-income students to pursue a postsecondary education. It will require political changes to reverse this dynamic.

The lack of low-income housing is a serious problem for individuals and families across the nation, and it is no different for MATC's students. The Milwaukee housing market, in particular, is in disequilibrium—there is a significant mismatch between the demand for low- and moderate-income housing and the supply. As a result, the rents for modest apartments in less-than-desirable neighborhoods remain unacceptably high. At the same time, there is a housing boom in downtown Milwaukee, where MATC's flagship campus is located. Like in many cities, these developments are often publically subsidized through tax increment financing districts, New Markets Tax Credits, and other forms of public support. But the rents are simply unaffordable for MATC's students. Milwaukee mayor Tom Barrett recently announced that the city had created almost 12,000 new residential units. But "just 760 of those new units, says Department of City Development commissioner Rocky Marcoux, are affordable."[38] Cities need to pursue ordinances that would require developers receiving public dollars to include a percentage of low- and moderate-income units. That would help ease the shortage of low- and moderate-income housing and, in Milwaukee, allow MATC students to obtain affordable housing in close proximity to where they attend classes.

At the same time, the work of the FAST Fund has helped expose smaller policy changes that could improve students' lives. The 150 percent credit rule for federal financial aid is too rigid. It frequently penalizes students who are simply trying to improve their skills and secure better jobs. For example, Diane is an MATC nursing student. A decade ago, she had used financial aid to pursue an associate degree in human services. After earning her degree and working in the field for several years, she decided to pursue a career change to become a nurse. She was accepted into the MATC nursing program but was no longer eligible for financial aid. Diane became a student who had to pay the full cost of her education.

Diane worked two full-time jobs prior to the beginning of her first semester in an effort to save money for school. When classes began, she left one job and became part-time in the other so she could concentrate on her studies. But with her reduced income, as she wrote to the FAST Fund, "I was only able to afford my rent, food and gas.

With the money I had saved I was only able to afford the books and classes."[39]

The MATC nursing program requires that students purchase an iPad from the college bookstore at a cost of roughly $520. It must be purchased through MATC because it is loaded with nursing-specific software. Despite her careful budgeting, Diane did not have sufficient funds to purchase the iPad. The FAST Fund stepped in and purchased it for her. But there is no legitimate reason a hard-working, low-income student like Diane should be denied public support. The denial is particularly egregious since Diane had been working and paying taxes that help pay for Pell Grants and other federal programs for almost a decade.

Education is a positive externality, meaning that the benefits accrue not just to the individual student but also to society more broadly. Diane's pursuit of a health nursing degree would benefit not only her but also future employers and patients since there is a shortage of nurses in Wisconsin, which is anticipated to grow even more severe.[40] Policymakers need to review the rules governing federal financial aid so that students like Diane who return to school to pursue additional degrees are supported in their efforts.

Diane's experience is all too common. Tiana, another MATC student, graduated from Bryant Stratton, a Milwaukee-based for-profit college, with a degree in criminal justice and a $70,000 debt. Like so many students who attend for-profit colleges, she was unable to land a job in her field of study. During the Great Recession, for-profit colleges and developers using them as anchor tenants descended on Milwaukee.[41] Thousands of students like Tiana who attended Everest College, Sanford Brown, ITT Tech, Bryant Stratton, Kaplan, and others maximized their financial aid in pursuit of degrees and the promise of future family-supporting employment. All too frequently they end up unemployed, with credits that do not transfer, huge debts, and broken dreams.[42]

Tiana enrolled in MATC's respiratory therapist program. Because she had exhausted her financial aid at Bryant Stratton, she was paying out of pocket for her MATC education. But when she began her clinicals, a requirement in the program, she had to reduce her work hours. She fell behind on her rent. The FAST Fund provided her with a grant so she could keep her apartment. Tiana and others like her—students who have been victimized by fraudulent diploma mills but are working hard to escape poverty—should not be prevented by the 150 percent credit rule from furthering their education.

There are also federal regulations that at least some financial aid offices interpret as requiring emergency aid to count against a students' federal financial aid package. In some cases, students are even denied support because they have maxed out their financial aid for the semester. It is well established that Pell Grants and other sources of aid do not cover the total cost of college.[43] That is one reason why student debt has become the second-largest source of indebtedness in the United States.[44] Deducting emergency grants from an already-insufficient total allocation only makes matters worse. This harmful policy needs to be changed.

Pell Grants should also be substantially increased. As Goldrick-Rab has documented, "When the Pell program began, Pell Grants subsidized more than 80 percent of the cost of attending the average public university and all of the costs of attending a community college. Things are different now. Today the maximum Pell program covers less than one-third of the cost of attending a public four-year public university and barely 60 percent of the cost of attending a community college."[45]

Closer to home, there are several changes that MATC should make to assist low-income students, but the underlying concepts behind these recommendations likely apply to many colleges and universities across the United States.

The first point is about ensuring timely access to resources. Dreamkeepers is MATC's principal emergency assistance program. But when classes began in the fall of 2018, it was not open. It did not begin operations until September 24, a full month after classes had begun. It is also closed during the summer, despite the fact that thousands of students attend summer school, and during semester breaks. But poverty does not take semester or summer breaks. MATC's student needs are not aligned with the academic calendar. Dreamkeepers should remain open year-round.

In addition, MATC does not distribute financial aid checks until more than five weeks after a semester begins. The practice by MATC's and other colleges' financial aid offices of delaying the distribution of financial aid imposes an unnecessary economic hardship on students who count on their financial aid as a main source of income to pay for the full cost of college attendance. As a result of this practice, many MATC students are unable to pay their rent at the beginning of the semester. But when they apply to Dreamkeepers for assistance, they are refused because rent is not considered an unexpected expense. So these students contact the FAST Fund. Other colleges and universities distribute financial aid checks when their semesters begin. The money belongs not to the colleges but to the students. It should be distributed to the students at the beginning of the semester. Until MATC corrects this practice, Dreamkeepers should recognize that MATC students' need for housing support is a legitimate need and fund their requests. MATC's late disbursement practice also places undue pressure on the FAST Fund. The fund has limited dollars. When it uses dollars to assist students whose problems are the creation of MATC's bureaucracy, the opportunity cost is that those dollars are not available to address other students' needs.

Second is the related issue of physical location and access to resources. Last year, MATC established the Student Resource Center. The admirable purpose was to establish a single location where students could access a variety of services. But the center was located in a building that is not centrally located. In fact, no college classes are held in that building, and as a result, very few students sought services even when they were offered. The lack of student traffic was a result of the center's location rather than a lack of need. The FAST Fund directly served more than 100 students in 2017–18, and

Dreamkeepers helped an additional 259 students, but it denied 475 students who applied and were in need of assistance but did not meet certain criteria. At least one agency that housed staff at the center said that they would have a hard time justifying allocating staff there again since it is not easily accessible to students. The Hunger Task Force had the same experience. To reach more students, their staff frequently set up a table in the MATC Student Center. If the expertise of students and faculty had been included in the planning process for the Student Resource Center, this access problem could have been avoided and it could have served more students.

Amarillo College, as explained in chapter 9 of this book, took an entirely different approach by locating their Advocacy and Resource Center (ARC) on the first floor, surrounded by windows, in its renovated Student Commons Building at the center of its main campus. While some staff worried that students would feel too exposed to use the ARC because of its location, this was not the case: "Demand for the ARC's services has grown dramatically. Herrera, the social services director, who presides over the ARC, believes the prime location has taken some of the stigma out of asking for help."[46] The MATC Student Resource Center is an important initiative. The college needs to reevaluate its location, with the help of students and faculty, in order to maximize its effectiveness in serving students.

Third, MATC and other colleges and universities should fund a student ombudsman position or positions to serve students in need. Currently the FAST Fund has played that role, trying to identify MATC and external resources to assist students in financial need. It would be far more effective if there were a dedicated employee with institutional authority and independence assigned this responsibility, as discussed in chapter 6 of this book.

Fourth, the education system must acknowledge and respond to the financial burden of clinical placements, internships, and practicum requirements. For example, MATC health science students are required to take clinicals as part of their education. But several students who contacted the FAST Fund explained that because clinicals are unpaid, their clinical participation reduced their income because they had to reduce their paid work hours. Colleges should explore the feasibility of partnering with hospitals to provide clinical compensation or establishing scholarships for students participating in clinicals.

Fifth, MATC, like many colleges, will not provide graduating students with transcripts if they owe the college money. But a transcript is almost always required for students to obtain employment. It is a self-defeating policy—a catch-22. The college's policy effectively prevents graduates from obtaining employment, but without a job the graduate will not be able to pay MATC back. The FAST Fund has successfully intervened to obtain an official transcript for indebted graduates on two occasions. It is antithetical to a technical college's mission to prevent its graduates from obtaining employment. Colleges need a more student-friendly, flexible policy.

Conclusion

The AFT Local 212/MATC FAST Fund's experience confirms the University of Wisconsin HOPE Lab's research that a principal obstacle to student retention and completion is economic insecurity. The need for additional resources is widespread.[47] If this need is not addressed, other popular student success strategies, such as guided pathways, will not be successful.

The FAST Fund is committed to continuing emergency support to MATC's students. To accomplish this goal, it will continue to raise funds from traditional sources of support while trying to expand fundraising to foundations and the philanthropic community. The AFT Local 212/MATC FAST Fund will use its experience to promote systemic and institutional change. The fund's director has been appointed to a city of Milwaukee commission on evictions, and faculty union leaders will advocate for the changes in federal financial aid and the MATC policies discussed earlier.

The FAST Fund's experience is clear—unless the nation addresses the economic needs of low- and moderate-income students, the nation will not make real progress in improving college completion rates, helping low- and moderate-income students gain a foothold in the middle class, or reducing inequality, which are all hurting our economy and undermining our democracy.

Notes

1. Rosalind Simmons, interview with author, Aug. 20, 2018.

2. "Federal Regulation 34 CFR § 668.34," Cornell University Legal Information Institute, https://www.law.cornell.edu/cfr/text/34/668.34.

3. "Dreamkeepers," Madison Area Technical College, https://matc.dreamkeepers.org/.

4. Kevin Crowe and Bill Glauber, "Wisconsin Incomes Up, Poverty Down," *Milwaukee Journal Sentinel*, Sept. 14, 2016, https://www.jsonline.com/story/news/2016/09/15/wisconsin-incomes-up-poverty-down/90355098/.

5. Matthew Desmond, *Evicted: Poverty and Profit in the American City* (New York: Crown, 2016), 24.

6. Barbara Miner, *Lessons from the Heartland* (New York: New Press, 2013), 114.

7. Marc Levine, *Perspectives on the Current State of the Milwaukee Economy* (Milwaukee: University of Wisconsin–Milwaukee, Center for Economic Development, July 2013), 8.

8. John Schmitt and Janelle Jones, "Bad Jobs on the Rise," *Center for Economic and Policy Research*, Sept. 2012, 1.

9. Levine, *Perspectives*, 21.

10. Desmond, *Evicted*, 24.

11. Jason De Perle, *American Dream: Three Women, Ten Kids, and a Nation's Drive to End Welfare* (London: Penguin Books, 2005), 61.

12. Levine, *Perspectives*, 18.

13. John Schmid, "A Dream Derailed: Hit by a Global Train," *Milwaukee Journal Sentinel*, Dec. 5–7, 2004, https://graphics.jsonline.com/jsi_news/projects/2004/A-Dream-Derailed.pdf.

14. Levine, *Perspectives*, 11.

15. Desmond, *Evicted*, 98.

16. Desmond, *Evicted*, 5.

17. Yan Wang, email to author, June 11, 2018.

18. See http://www.thefastfund.org/.

19. "The FAST Fund," Sara Goldrick-Rab (website), https:// saragoldrickrab.com/fastfund/.

20. Sara Goldrick-Rab, *Paying the Price: College Costs, Financial Aid, and the Betrayal of the American Dream* (Chicago: University of Chicago Press, 2016), 205–8.

21. Goldrick-Rab, *Paying the Price*, 193.

22. Karen Herzog, "Union Raises Almost $17,000 to Help MATC Students Facing Sudden Financial Crisis Stay in School," *Milwaukee Journal Sentinel*, July 28, 2017, https://www.jsonline.com/story/news/education /2017/07/28/union-raises-nearly-17-000-help-matc-students-facing -sudden-financial-crisis-stay-school/519794001/.

23. Sara Goldrick-Rab, "We're in This Together," *Medium*, Nov. 29, 2017, https://medium.com/@saragoldrickrab/were-in-this-together -52d582f088fa.

24. Desmond, *Evicted*, 98.

25. Jennifer Curlin, interview with author, Sept. 9, 2018.

26. Marcella Bombardieri, "Community Colleges Are No Match for American Poverty," *City Lab*, May 31, 2018, https://www.citylab.com/equity /2018/05/community-colleges-are-no-match-for-american-poverty /561596/.

27. Priscilla Rangel, email to author, Feb. 2, 2018.

28. Jessica Adkinson, email to author, Feb. 10, 2018.

29. "Last-dollar" and "first-dollar" are two distinct methods of distributing funding for college promise programs. Last-dollar program design means that students draw on any available public funding before being awarded any new college promise funds. First-dollar program design means that college promise funds are provided to students first, or before any other grant or awarded funding. See, e.g., https://www.acct.org/page/first-dollar -vs-last-dollar-promise-models.

30. Karen Herzog, "MATC Rolling Out New Free Tuition Program to Lure Working Adults Back to Finish College," *Milwaukee Journal Sentinel*, May 17, 2018, https://www.jsonline.com/story/news/education/2018/05/17 /matc-offering-free-tuition-eligible-adults-finish-college/609707002/.

31. Mareza Landeros, email to author, Sept. 12, 2018.

32. Josue Davalos, interview with author, July 25, 2018.

33. Student Satisfaction Inventory (SSI) Survey Results, MATC, Spring 2016.

34. Lee Fang and Nick Surgey, "Right-Wing, Business-Funded Groups Are Preparing to Use the Janus Decision to Bleed Unions, Internal Documents Show," *Intercept*, June 30, 2018, https://theintercept.com/2018/06/30 /janus-bleed-unions-state-policy-network/.

35. See http://www.thefastfund.org/.

36. Bill Glauber, "Study: In 2016, State's Job Market Improved, but Poverty Increased," *Milwaukee Journal Sentinel*, June 8, 2018, https://www .jsonline.com/story/news/politics/2018/06/08/2016-wisconsins-job -market-improved-but-poverty-rate-increased/679254002/.

37. Valarie Strauss, "Is Gov. Scott Walker Putting the University of Wisconsin System in Jeopardy?," *Washington Post*, June 5, 2015, https://www.washingtonpost.com/news/answer-sheet/wp/2015/06/05/is-gov-scott-walker-putting-the-university-of-wisconsin-system-in-jeopardy/?utm_term=.c2b3406f7433.

38. Susan Nusser, "Can Milwaukee Really Create 10,000 Affordable Homes?," *City Lab*, Oct. 22, 2018, https://www.citylab.com/equity/2018/10/can-milwaukee-really-create-10000-affordable-homes/570742/?fbclid=IwAR1Tj1orGhLYCUYoWFQaOo4ForXYo-vDogi-UCAqR8SVlYzmoejnX53BqPg.

39. Diane Thomas, email to author, Feb. 25, 2018.

40. Linda Young and Jan Adams, "Nursing Faculty Shortage in Wisconsin: Impact on Nursing Workforce," *University of Wisconsin–Eau Claire College of Nursing and Health Sciences*, Dec. 2015, https://wisconsinnurses.org/wp-content/uploads/2015/12/Faculty-Shortage-_L-Young.pdf.

41. Joel Dresang, "Milwaukee's For-Profit Colleges Doing Well during the Recession," *Milwaukee Journal Sentinel*, Aug. 28, 2009, http://archive.jsonline.com/business/55949037.html/.

42. Associated Press, "Almost All Student Loan Fraud Claims Involve For-Profit Colleges, Study Finds," *Los Angeles Times*, Nov. 9, 2017, http://www.latimes.com/business/la-fi-student-loan-forgiveness-20171109-story.html.

43. Goldrick-Rab, *Paying the Price*, 52.

44. Jessica Dickler, "Student Loan Balances Jump Nearly 150 Percent in a Decade," *CNBC*, Aug. 29, 2017, https://www.cnbc.com/2017/08/29/student-loan-balances-jump-nearly-150-percent-in-a-decade.html.

45. Goldrick-Rab, *Paying the Price*, 17.

46. Bombardieri, "Community Colleges."

47. Sara Goldrick-Rab et al., *Still Hungry and Homeless in College* (Madison: Wisconsin HOPE Lab, 2018), https://hope4college.com/wp-content/uploads/2018/09/Wisconsin-HOPE-Lab-Still-Hungry-and-Homeless.pdf. For more information, see https://hope4college.com.

[4]

Channeling Student Idealism and Energy through Campus Organizing

TALIA BERDAY-SACKS AND JAMES DUBICK

Editors' Prologue. College students have long played a crucial role in drawing attention to social injustices and advocating for the rights and needs of those who are marginalized. In many ways, students are at the heart of the current movement to end hunger on college campuses. This chapter examines the growth of student activism around campus food insecurity, with a focus on two student-driven organizations working to address it: Challah for Hunger (CfH), an international nonprofit that equips and inspires communities to address hunger, and the National Student Campaign Against Hunger and Homelessness (NSCAHH), a campus network that promotes service, education, and advocacy regarding hunger and homelessness. The authors include examples of student action to address campus hunger, using these two organizations' approaches, to highlight lessons and recommendations for professionals and student activists on how to build a robust student movement around the issue of hunger on college campuses.

About the Authors. Talia Berday-Sacks managed Challah for Hunger's campus program from 2015 to 2018. Her passion for advocacy, food justice, and community empowerment began when she was an undergraduate volunteer for the Challah for Hunger chapter at the University of Maryland. She oversaw volunteer engagement, campaign planning, and partnership development for the Campus Hunger Project, a national advocacy initiative addressing college food insecurity.

James Dubick has a long career in student organizing, beginning as a campus organizer with the Student Public Interest Research Groups in 1999. He was the director of the National Student Campaign Against Hunger and Homelessness from 2014 to 2018. He is the coauthor of *Hunger on Campus: The Challenge of Food Insecurity for College Students,* a multicampus study on student hunger.[1]

The Role of Campus Activism in Social Change

To understand the potential power of campus activism to end student hunger, it is important to place this new movement in the context of past student activism. From civil rights to free speech, to feminism, to environmentalism, college students have been at the forefront of many major social movements of the past century. Students have the power to engage society in critical dialogues about urgent problems, amplify the voices of underrepresented communities, and ultimately change policies for the better.

Student activism has existed for nearly as long as the modern university. An early instance of coordinated student action took place in the 1930s, when students formed advocacy organizations such as the American Youth Congress (AYC) in response to the Great Depression and the impending threat of war. The AYC brought together hundreds of student and youth organizations from around the country to lobby for education spending, racial justice, and economic programs targeted at youth.[2] Their work won the support of Eleanor Roosevelt, who was deeply concerned at the time about the need to increase civic engagement among young people.[3] Another historic example is Berkeley's free speech movement in the 1960s, when student protests forced the University of California to acknowledge students' right to engage in political speech on campus, paving the way for every student movement that came afterward.[4]

The civil rights movement is a commonly recognized demonstration of the power of college students. The campus movement to end segregation began in earnest in 1960 when students from North Carolina A&T College sat in at the Woolworth's lunch counter in Greensboro, North Carolina. Their actions inspired similar sit-ins throughout the South.[5] The student leaders forged by those events went on to create the Student Nonviolent Coordinating Committee (SNCC), which became one of the leading civil rights organizations of the 1960s. In 1964, SNCC helped organize Freedom Summer, one of the most famous projects from that period, which brought more than 1,000 college students to Mississippi to register black voters.[6]

That same desire to end inequality drove the campus anti-apartheid movement two decades later. Students joined the movement by calling for their colleges to divest from companies that traded with or had operations in South Africa. Campus protests drew attention to South Africa's institutional system of racial discrimination, while also putting financial pressure on the South African government. Student actions convinced more than 150 colleges and universities to divest.[7] Years later, Nelson Mandela asserted that the University of California's decision to divest billions of dollars in investments from South Africa had a significant impact on ending apartheid.[8]

Student Activism to End Poverty

The movement to end hunger and homelessness is no exception to these historical trends. Students have consistently played a role here as well. This student movement took off in the 1980s, when the rapid expansion of visible homelessness in American cities inspired a wave of activism to tackle poverty.[9] Some students joined advocacy campaigns to lobby for public programs to alleviate hunger and homelessness, while others turned to direct service as a solution by volunteering in soup kitchens or organizing food and clothing drives. Service-based organizations like Habitat for Humanity set up chapters on many campuses.[10]

During the 1980s, a highly publicized African famine also drove new interest among students around global hunger. For many college students, Hands Across America was their first introduction to the fight against poverty. On May 25, 1986, seven million people linked hands to form a human chain from New York City to Los Angeles.[11] Countless students, from kindergarten through college, joined the event to raise money and awareness about global poverty.

Anti-hunger activism also benefited from a movement within the higher education community during the 1980s and 1990s to incorporate civic engagement and community service as essential aspects of the educational experience. Service-learning programs, which incorporate community service into classroom studies, spread rapidly.[12] Many colleges opened new offices to promote service and engagement and manage new programs like freshman orientation service projects and Alternative Spring Break. The Campus Opportunity Outreach League was created in 1984 to connect this new community of campus organizations and administrators devoted to community engagement.[13] A year later, university presidents launched Campus Compact, an organization that supports college administrators in making community engagement an institutional priority.[14]

These waves of anti-hunger activism, along with the academic community's investment in civic engagement and service learning, gave students powerful ways to engage in the movement to end poverty. Over time, campus activism around poverty and inequality expanded to take on many forms, including widely publicized campaigns to end the use of sweatshop labor for university products and pay campus workers a living wage.[15] Some students directed their activism inward by working to change their own campuses' policies on issues such as mental health, sexual assault, and racial and gender equality and inclusion. For college students, campus is their home and community, and they are constantly seeking ways to improve it.

Addressing Student Food Insecurity

Over the past five years there has been a growing awareness among students about food insecurity on their campuses, impacting themselves or their peers. This problem exists in the context of long-simmering debates over income inequality, diversity, and inclusion in higher education. There has been a concerted push by colleges and universities to admit and retain more students from historically marginalized and underrepresented groups, but schools have not always done enough to meet the needs of their changing student bodies. The combination of a more socioeconomically diverse student population and rapidly rising costs has created the conditions for a campus hunger crisis.[16] This issue has become particularly compelling for students who feel a personal connection to the problem because they are food insecure themselves or have friends who experience this challenge.

Established anti-hunger movements have found success because of robust networks of activist organizations that provide students with issue expertise and campaign direction. However, until recently there was not an existing community of activist groups with the capacity to train and lead students who wanted to address campus hunger. Numerous groups have emerged in recent years that have begun to fill that vacuum, including the College and University Food Bank Alliance, Swipe Out Hunger, the Campus Kitchens Project, and the Food Recovery Network.

This section looks at the ways in which two nonprofit organizations—Challah for Hunger (CfH) and the National Student Campaign Against Hunger and Homelessness (NSCAHH)—have recruited, trained, and mobilized college students to address student food insecurity. These national organizations have taken distinctly different approaches to mobilizing college students owing to their different organizational structures, priorities, and student engagement models, but their combined work on more than 200 campuses provides lessons on how to support and promote activism around student food insecurity.

CfH and NSCAHH

CfH has been working with college students since 2004, when Eli Winkelman, a student at Scripps College, started the organization to build community and awareness about the genocide in Darfur. Her idea quickly spread, and now CfH serves thousands of students annually on more than 80 college campuses. Since then, CfH has shifted their focus to addressing hunger and food insecurity, including recent efforts to address hunger among students on campus.[17]

At CfH chapters, student volunteers come together to bake challah bread. While dough rises, they discuss local and global hunger issues and advocacy tactics. They then sell the challah to fellow students, university staff, and community members. Fifty percent of their profits are donated to MAZON: A Jewish Response to Hunger, and 50 percent to a local nonprofit fighting hunger in their community. Since 2004, CfH volunteers have donated more than $1 million to hunger relief and social justice nonprofits. In addition to providing students with resources and support to run the daily operations of a social enterprise—a bread bakery—CfH provides extensive training in volunteer management, responsible philanthropy, partnership development, and advocacy. CfH also guides chapters in developing and implementing campaigns to raise awareness of food insecurity and advocate for long-term solutions.

NSCAHH was created in 1985 to increase student community service and advocacy to end hunger and homelessness by offering resources, support, and guidance to college students across the country. As famine swept across Ethiopia in the early 1980s, threatening millions of people with starvation, countless Americans felt compelled by this crisis happening on the other side of the world to take action. Recognizing the incredible potential of the collective power of young people, USA for Africa and the Public Interest Research Groups combined their resources to establish NSCAHH. In its first few years, NSCAHH raised more than $250,000 for hunger relief through its "Let's Start Giving Campaign," collected 85,000 signatures to encourage decision-makers to "Stamp Out Hunger," helped organize millions of Americans to join in "Hands Across America," and surveyed emergency food recipients for a research report titled "Portrait of America's Hungry."[18]

Developing Leaders: CfH's Campus Hunger Project

In 2016, CfH launched a campaign called the Campus Hunger Project to investigate food insecurity on campuses with CfH chapters, educate the wider CfH community about this issue, and develop a strategy for supporting food-insecure students. In its first year, the Campus Hunger Project had an educational focus. With support from staff and a student advisory committee, students from 23 universities gathered information about food insecurity on their campuses through 32 interviews with university administrators. Students found that approximately 80 percent of administrators recognized that food insecurity was a problem on their campus, but of these administrators, 65 percent said that there was no official policy to address the issue. The types of emergency aid available to students, including food pantries, meal vouchers, and emergency grants or loans, varied greatly from institution to institution, as did methods for disseminating information about the availability of aid. Perhaps most notable, administrators' knowledge of aid programs and of procedures and policies for connecting students to aid programs varied as well.[19]

In its first year, the Campus Hunger Project also provided tools for students to raise awareness about campus hunger. Students could subscribe to a bimonthly email digest of research into the root causes of college food insecurity and were encouraged to share what they learned on social media. Students also had access to a digital toolkit with news articles, fact sheets, and discussion guides that they could use to learn about the issue individually or collectively as a chapter. As of early fall 2018, CfH had engaged students on 53 campuses with the Campus Hunger Project.

Findings from the interview project led CfH to make programmatic changes within the Campus Hunger Project in the second and third years of the campaign. The resources and policies in place on campuses varied too much to make a single recommendation to CfH volunteers on how to help food-insecure students get the support they need. Feedback from volunteers also revealed that students would need to be trained in organizing and advocacy skills if they were going to lead successful campaigns to change campus policies.

Based on these conclusions, CfH decided to focus their efforts on training 10 student representatives each year to run targeted campaigns specific to the needs of their individual campuses. Through a nine-month leadership development program called the Campus Hunger Project Cohort, students learn about campus food insecurity from experts in the field and then plan and execute campaigns to change campus policies. The Cohort launches each year with an in-person gathering, followed by monthly curriculum-based virtual trainings where students develop core advocacy and organizing skills. Throughout the program, students receive individual coaching from a dedicated staff member and are provided with funding to use toward their campaign and for additional professional development. For example, students have used this funding for Facebook advertising, event space rental, and campaign marketing materials. To enable students from all backgrounds to participate, travel for the in-person gathering is fully funded by CfH, and students receive a stipend for the time they invest in the program.

Students in the 2017–18 Cohort took creative and varied approaches to mobilizing their peers and campus communities around food insecurity. Diego and Lauren, Cohort members at the University of Wisconsin–Madison, organized workshops to train student government representatives to become peer advocates for food-insecure students. Gadi, a Cohort member at Temple University, raised more than $15,000 to support their new campus food pantry and organized an event to celebrate the pantry's launch that featured Dr. Sara Goldrick-Rab, the nation's leading expert on college food insecurity, as a speaker. Rachel from the University of Southern California advocated for professors in the College of Education to include information about emergency food and housing resources in their class syllabi. Hana from the University of California, Davis, served on a student-faculty task force that launched the Aggie Compass Basic Needs Center, a new service to point students toward resources to help fulfill basic needs like food, housing, and financial wellness.

The Cohort members were asked to reflect on the experience in their own words:

Participating in the Cohort has empowered me to be an advocate in my community. I see myself as an advocate in a way I certainly hadn't before, and believe I am now likely to continue working to reduce food insecurity throughout my life.

—Hana, University of California, Davis

Participating in the Cohort has allowed me to define my role as an advocate on the UW-Madison campus. It has made my entire experience with Challah for Hunger much more meaningful, because it allowed me to feel as though one person has the power to enact change on campus even if it is only within a small group. The Cohort also connected me with a group of students who have provided invaluable advice and support.

—Lauren, University of Wisconsin–Madison

Beyond equipping students to engage in advanced advocacy tactics, an intended outcome of the Cohort is to inspire other volunteers to see advocacy as an inseparable function of their chapter's work. CfH is now investing additional time and resources to grow the Cohort and further integrate advocacy trainings into chapters' service and philanthropy programs. The goal in doing so is to strengthen the campus activist movement around college food insecurity and empower students to be more effective in seeking social change, both on campus and in their post-educational careers.

Raising Awareness: NSCAHH's Hunger and Homelessness Awareness Week

Shortly after its inception, NSCAHH became the national cosponsor, along with the National Coalition for the Homeless, of Hunger and Homelessness Awareness Week (HHAW). HHAW takes place each November during the week prior to Thanksgiving and brings public attention to the difficulties faced by people who are experiencing hunger and homelessness, fosters greater understanding and solidarity for those in need, and mobilizes people to act. NSCAHH organizes college campuses to participate, while the National Coalition for the Homeless organizes shelters, food banks, churches, and other community organizations.

The first HHAW was held at Villanova University in 1975. Since then, the event has grown dramatically, with an estimated 200 colleges and universities working to draw attention to the pressing issues of hunger and homelessness. Each participating campus designs their own schedule of events to hold during HHAW, typically including a mix of educational programs, community service activities, fundraisers, and advocacy projects. In the process, they engage tens of thousands of students and reach an audience of millions.

HHAW is designed to cast a wide net to involve as many people as possible. While some organizing projects are focused on going deep—working with a small number of very committed activists to develop them into powerful leaders—HHAW is designed to go broad. The program does provide opportunities to develop leaders— in fact, the students and community members who lead their local HHAW events build skills and become stronger activists through the experience—but the program's mission is to involve a wide range of people and groups and maximize its educational impact on participants and the public. The ideal HHAW brings together students, organizations, faculty members, administrators, local businesses, and local agencies and uses mainstream media, social media, publicity, and face-to-face outreach to reach the widest possible audience.

The most recent HHAW at the University of California, Berkeley, demonstrates the power of this program. The week was organized by the Berkeley Basic Needs Security Committee, which was created as part of a University of California system-wide initiative to address student food and housing insecurity. The committee organized an impressive week of events, with an estimated 4,000 Berkeley students attending HHAW events or participating in HHAW activities.

The largest event of the week was a "CalFresh mega clinic," where nearly 200 students sat down with volunteers from the Alameda County Food Bank, who helped them fill out applications for CalFresh, the state's program for providing Supplemental Nutrition Assistance Program (SNAP) benefits. In the campus dining halls, volunteers raised awareness about food waste by having students dump their leftovers into huge bins, so they could see firsthand the amount of food being thrown away. The committee also held a resource fair for low-income students; workshops on mental health issues and on financial aid; a community dinner; a panel discussion including speakers from Congresswoman Barbara Lee's office, the Berkeley Food Institute, and the student government; and a competition where students were challenged to see who could make the best proposal for how to reduce the barriers to entry that discourage students from applying for CalFresh benefits.

The week was coordinated by Sara, a Berkeley sophomore. Sara first became involved with the Basic Needs Security Committee as a first-year student by volunteering with the campus food pantry. At the end of the year, Sara applied for and became the committee's community programs coordinator, a paid leadership position. Planning HHAW gave Sara the opportunity to tackle her largest leadership role to date. For HHAW, she led four interns and a team of volunteers as they planned the week's events, creating a budget, setting up logistics, and liaising with other organizations. For the coming year, she plans to lead HHAW again, with goals to engage even more partners at her college and collaborate with students organizing HHAW events at other University of California campuses. Sara described the experience as follows:

Organizing Berkeley's campaign for HHAW has been one of the most meaningful and challenging experiences I've had. Through the process of planning holistic programming that addressed the intersections of basic needs security with other social issues, I was able to partner with experts who are doing truly amazing work in their respective fields and learn about the gaps that still exist. It was really interesting to hear from the different perspectives among the campus community and see how our programming provoked people to continue the dialogue beyond the duration of the campaign. Though exhausting, this experience has been incredible, and I can't wait to build upon this success next year.

In total, 2017's HHAW involved more than 1,000 local organizations in 400 communities. Thirty-five nonprofits participated as national partners in the event, publicizing it to their networks. The week's events were covered in hundreds of local media stories and generated millions of impressions on social media.

Lessons Learned

Through these experiences, CfH and NSCAHH have field-tested different approaches to campus organizing, providing insight on how to most effectively recruit student volunteers, develop student leaders, and evaluate success. The accomplishments and challenges of these programs provide valuable lessons on how to design future programs and campaigns for maximum impact.

Recruiting Student Activists

CfH and NSCAHH recruit and train students throughout the school year, building a pipeline of volunteers to participate in their programs. To build a strong volunteer base, campus organizations like these must design programs that appeal to a wide range of students. Service events like CfH's weekly challah baking event tend to have the broadest appeal since they have the lowest barrier to entry and are ideal for students who want an accessible way to make an impact while also enjoying the social aspect of volunteering with a group. However, programs should offer opportunities designed to appeal to the many different motivations that potential volunteers have for getting involved, including giving back to their communities, building professional skills, gaining leadership experience, and bonding with other students.

While community service activities are powerful tools for recruitment, this should not discourage groups from pursuing advocacy programs to seek policy reforms and systemic change. For many students, repeated exposure to service and educational activities can inspire a desire to tackle larger challenges. Hands-on experience at programs like a food pantry can deepen students' understanding of an issue and its systemic causes and motivate them to seek long-term solutions. Campus leaders and staffers can foster this process by moving students up a ladder of engagement, encouraging them to take on increasing levels of responsibility and leadership. If groups fail to provide these opportunities, they may lose advocacy-minded students to other organizations.

Recruitment can often be difficult, no matter the program. Volunteer opportunities compete with the countless other options that students have for how to spend their time. Classes, jobs, other organizations, and personal obligations all make it challenging for students to join new programs that come with a large time commitment. To overcome this, it is important to constantly be recruiting and inviting new students to become involved.

For example, CfH initially struggled to recruit students to participate in the Campus Hunger Project. CfH staff members primarily communicate with the executive leaders in each chapter, those who handle the day-to-day responsibilities of running the group. These students are deeply committed, handling the chapter's finances, marketing, and volunteer management and often taking on added responsibilities like helping plan CfH's annual leadership conference. While these highly involved students expressed initial excitement about the Cohort, many hesitated to commit to yet another time-intensive project. To solve this challenge, staff members began closely monitoring CfH's online volunteer engagement platform and following up individually by phone or email with students who interacted with any of the Campus Hunger Project's online resources. In this way, CfH staffers were able to build new relationships with students who had not previously been chapter leaders but who demonstrated interest in advocacy-focused opportunities.

For HHAW, NSCAHH frequently takes advantage of existing campus systems to assist with recruitment. At many schools, NSCAHH works with campus administrators in departments like student activities, civic engagement, or volunteerism who are tasked with promoting student involvement. These administrators have existing relationships with student activists, access to campus marketing channels, and funding to subsidize programs. By reaching out to these campus staff members and enlisting them to support HHAW, NSCAHH develops liaisons on campus who can use the school's own resources to recruit interested students to become HHAW leaders.

Training a Wide-Ranging Volunteer Base

Regional and national student activist organizations often find it challenging to manage their widespread volunteer base. Opportunities to train and build meaningful relationships with volunteers in person are often limited owing to logistical constraints. For this reason, organizations with professional staff tend to invest time in developing downloadable toolkits, webinars, and other online resources.

A growing number of campus-based organizations, including CfH, manage and mobilize volunteers through an online platform developed by the Enlight Foundation. Originally developed under the foundation's Crew2030 initiative, the Enlight platform is a tool for training volunteers in an interactive learning environment.[20] The platform transformed how CfH trains students to operate and strengthen their chapters. Before using the platform, staff shared organizational policies, educational resources, and reporting tools through lengthy handbooks that were created and edited by the organization's alumni. However, the handbooks existed in physical and digital forms that were sometimes difficult to share. After implementing the Enlight platform in 2015, staffers migrated over a decade's worth of resources into a user-friendly online library and training center.

The platform uses a "gamification" strategy to motivate students to complete trainings and engage with educational and advocacy campaigns like the Campus Hunger Project. Students complete preset learning modules featuring short webinars, articles, and reflection questions and receive positive reinforcement in the form of points and badges. Points can then be spent in a virtual store that offers marketing materials and funding for event supplies. For CfH's geographically distributed network of volunteers, the platform also allows students to share their accomplishments with their peers and enables staffers to track how often individual resources are used. Most importantly, the platform helps staffers identify students who make the most use of the platform and recruit them for leadership opportunities like the Cohort.

Technologies like this platform can streamline the training process for volunteers, fueling deeper engagement with organizations' programs and educational resources. However, remote learning does have drawbacks, especially for lessons that focus on building an individual's interpersonal skills. In addition, in-person training has built-in mechanisms for feedback. If an in-person training is not connecting with trainees, the trainer can see that and adjust accordingly. If participants have questions, there is room within an in-person training to easily discuss them. Online training methods do not always have the same feedback mechanisms.

CfH faced this challenge when they published a digital advocacy toolkit on the Enlight platform. The toolkit outlined three ways for volunteers to participate in the Campus Hunger Project: completing a training module about the root causes and impacts of student food insecurity, gathering data on the issue through online research and one-on-one interviews with campus administrators, and leading an interactive group discussion with their CfH chapter about the project. Many volunteers struggled to implement the program, and the reason only became clear when CfH staff solicited students' feedback. Although each step of the program built on the one before, students' responses revealed that many were not implementing the program activities in their designated order because the toolkit had not made the sequence clear. The organization tested new online layouts and instructions for each activity, which solved this problem.

For far-flung student networks, conferences can provide an opportunity to provide advanced training in person. For twenty years, NSCAHH organized an annual conference that brought together hundreds of student leaders to discuss their work to end hunger and homelessness. The conference featured workshops where students could learn about a wide range of issues and skills from experts in the field. In addition, the conference's Opportunities and Action Fair featured exhibits staffed by national anti-poverty organizations where students could learn how to get involved in their programs. Along with the opportunity to gain knowledge and skills, conferences can also inspire and motivate student leaders by helping them see the full scope of the movement and feed off the group energy of the event.

While conferences can be powerful training experiences, they require months of planning and recruitment. The huge amount of work involved discourages many organizations from holding them, particularly smaller organizations with limited resources. In addition, it is important for conferences to provide scholarships for attendees who need assistance with travel or other expenses, in order to make these events accessible for everyone.

Evaluating Impact

Another challenge with running a widely distributed network arises when trying to evaluate programs and measure their impact. Careful data collection and self-evaluation are critical so that organizations can assess their efforts and plan effectively. However, the students running these programs on campus typically have no formal accountability to the national organization. As volunteers, they choose when and how to participate in programs. As a result, it can be difficult to get them to submit timely qualitative or quantitative updates on their work and accomplishments.

CfH's online platform attempts to address this by embedding polls and surveys directly into online training modules, giving students the opportunity to self-reflect before too much time elapses. The platform also rewards students with points and positive feedback when they submit reports after completing certain modules, providing incentives that increase their likelihood of doing so. When students fail to complete these modules, CfH staffers personally reach out to students to encourage their completion.

One way that NSCAHH attempts to mitigate this challenge is by formalizing students' responsibilities to their programs. On some campuses, student leaders can treat their work with NSCAHH as an internship or independent study course. To successfully complete the internship or course, students need to complete a set of predetermined requirements, including regularly reporting their work product. Similarly, some universities' student activities departments are able to hire student leaders as part-time staff and pay them to plan and support campus activities like HHAW, making data collection and reporting part of their job.

Building the Campus Hunger Movement

In order for the student movement to end campus hunge.
come fully realized, it will need to build a robust infrastru
to support and foster student activists. For an understanding of
what this will entail, this section presents a set of recommendations gleaned from CfH's and NSCAHH's programs and other campus movements to guide student activists and professionals who
support student activism.

Put Students at the Center of the Movement

It might not be immediately clear why student activism is a necessary part of the movement to address student food insecurity. One
could argue that this is a problem that could be solved by higher education leaders, campus administrators, and policy experts. While
their support is essential for ending student hunger and homelessness, these stakeholders are only part of the solution.

Any movement that wants to achieve social change needs to involve the community most affected by the problem. As the affected
population, students understand the challenges of their own food
insecurity better than anyone, so their input is crucial to developing interventions that will succeed. Students are the ones experiencing the problem, so they are best situated to come up with creative
solutions. In addition, students are the best messengers for those solutions, as students are more likely to accept and utilize programs
that are designed, endorsed, and recommended by their peers. Ultimately, colleges cannot solve this problem *for* students. They need
to solve it *with* students.

Student activists involved in the current high-profile drive to prevent campus sexual assault have shown the power of this approach.
For example, Know Your IX, one of the leading groups in the movement, was founded by sexual assault survivors from Amherst College and Yale Law School to serve as a survivor-led voice to end

sexual violence on campuses.[21] The organization consists of current students and recent graduates who provide support and training to student survivors as they demand institutional changes from their college administrations. In doing so, they help ensure that students have a voice in how their colleges address this issue.

Campus administrators and nonprofits need to make sure that students are fully represented in discussions about campus hunger. When decisions are being made about programs to address campus food insecurity, student leaders need to be in the room and have an equal voice. In addition, students need to be given space and encouragement to create their own student-led efforts to find solutions.

Bring Everyone to the Table

Powerful movements are ones that find a way to develop a broad base that is inclusive of the entire community. This requires organizations to identify challenges that might limit involvement and develop strategies to address them. For students whose basic needs are not being met, it can be hard to find the time, energy, and resources to be an activist. Volunteer programs can be a strain on the schedules and budgets of working students, student parents, and others who face a higher risk of food insecurity. Community service projects often take place during the evening or on weekends and conflict with some students' work schedules or need to provide childcare. Big events like conferences, lobby days, and leadership trainings can present even larger scheduling challenges. In addition, these large events can be expensive for participants, with costs for travel, housing, and registration fees.

Programs to end campus hunger need to actively involve students of all kinds, particularly but not limited to students who are directly experiencing these problems. When these students are missing from the spaces where conversations about solutions and strategies take place, these efforts risk alienating or even harming the very people they seek to help. Moreover, if food-insecure students are missing from these discussions, it can send a message to policymakers and university administrators that this problem is not important to students and does not need to be taken seriously.

An example of how student activism can strive to be inclusive of the voices of all students is the youth-led March for Our Lives. The event organizers recognized their own privileged position and made a concerted effort to include people of all backgrounds in their message about ending gun violence. The stories told by student leaders from Marjory Stoneman Douglas High School in Parkland, Florida, were at the heart of the march's message, but these students used their platform to speak out repeatedly about the need to address gun violence in every community, not just in their own relatively affluent suburb.[22] They reached out to students around the country to better understand how gun violence affected other schools and then made sure that the march featured a diverse range of speakers, including students from inner-city schools in Chicago, Los Angeles, and Washington, DC.[23] As the organization continues to expand following the march, there is more that they will need to do to be truly inclusive, but they have taken critical first steps by acknowledging the need for diversity within their movement and by pursuing steps to achieve it.

Organizations in the campus hunger movement need to determine the best ways to make their programs accessible to all and consider ways to remove barriers that might discourage participation by students from varying socioeconomic backgrounds. This starts with developing recruitment and marketing plans that target a wide range of students and partnering with organizations that serve underrepresented student groups. Groups can also promote an inclusive environment by creating flexible scheduling options for volunteers, providing subsidies or scholarships to cover expenses like supplies and travel, and creating paid positions through work-study programs to alleviate the opportunity cost between volunteering and employment.

Build a Collaborative Community

A strong movement to end campus food insecurity will require a robust community of regional and national organizations that can provide local students with the resources and support to make the most of their efforts. Community provides the structure to facilitate student activism. In addition, organizations provide a much-needed means for students to connect across campuses. This networking can come in many forms, including electronic communication such as email lists and texting groups, as well as in-person events such as regional and national conferences. These interactions are critical to movement growth, since they allow students to share ideas and provide each other with emotional support and inspiration.

The campus environmental movement provides a template for how this can look. Student environmental activists have a wide range of organizations with which they can affiliate, including the Sierra Student Coalition, 350.org, the National Wildlife Federation, the Rainforest Action Network, and the Public Interest Research Groups. No matter their specific interests, students can find an organization that fits their needs and shares their outlook. Having a wide range of groups provides the campus environmental movement with the breadth and depth to grow and sustain itself.

In addition, despite their differences, these organizations coordinate their efforts or collaborate on large projects when their interests overlap. For example, student organizations worked together to ensure that youth made up one of the core constituencies at the 2017 People's Climate March.[24] The march drew an estimated 200,000 marchers for the Washington, DC, event and thousands more at 300 events in other cities to demand solutions to climate change. The DC event even held a youth convening on the day before the march and a youth after-party after the event to bring together young participants.

Campus organizations like CfH, Swipe Out Hunger, and the Campus Kitchens Project have coordinated action on different campuses with their programs. Swipe Out Hunger helps students form partnerships with their campus dining center to donate meal swipes, and the Campus Kitchens Project recovers and donates food that would have otherwise gone to waste, often giving the food to students or campus pantries. In spite of these groups engaging in food insecurity alleviation work, the campus hunger movement does not yet have a formal coalition for coordinating programs. The movement needs to develop more robust systems for coordinating action between student groups working on the same campuses, in the same states, and across the country. Future partnerships could come in many forms. At the campus level, student coalitions could lobby individual administrators and university leadership for stronger support programs. On the state level, students at community colleges and four-year public institutions could combine forces to collectively lobby their lawmakers to change state policies around financial aid and SNAP. In addition to creating their own coalitions, student organizations also need to engage with existing anti-hunger coalitions established by the Food Research and Action Center, Feeding America, and MAZON: A Jewish Response to Hunger.

Develop Engaging Programs

When students decide they want to take on an issue like campus hunger, they often look for existing programs that they can bring to their own campus. For many students, creating their own program from scratch is a daunting task. Professional staff and campus administrators can remove this barrier by providing students with predesigned programs that they can easily pick up and implement.

One example of a long-running program with a proven track record of success is the Dance Marathon program, organized by the Children's Miracle Network Hospitals. Since Indiana University held the first event in 1991, dance marathons have spread to more than 300 colleges and universities in the United States and Canada and raised more than $200 million for pediatric hospitals.[25] The program gives students a well-tested model for planning the marathon and provides a clear way to mobilize their friends, families, and wider communities to support local charities. The program is easy for each campus to adapt to their needs—the main requirement is having a physical space where attendees can dance, play games, and socialize—and supports a popular cause.

The Interfaith Youth Core (IFYC) is another national nonprofit that provides students and educators with easy-to-adopt programming. IFYC partners with colleges and universities to turn religious diversity into a positive force in American society. They offer a host of program templates for students, including their "Talk Better Together" group dialogues and "speedfaithing" events, both of which are designed to help students of different faiths discuss their shared values and educate each other about their religions.[26]

The campus hunger movement has already begun down this path. Beyond CfH and NSCAHH, campus groups such as the Campus Kitchens Project, Swipe Out Hunger, and the Food Recovery Network (another campus-based food recovery program) have developed community service and philanthropic programs that students can pick up and run on their campuses. Each program offers a different model for reducing food insecurity, raising awareness, and becoming an advocate. For this movement to grow, new programs must emerge so that students have as many choices as possible for how to engage with this issue.

Build Leadership Pipelines

Grassroots movements need leaders, and student movements are no exception. However, most students do not come to college with activist experience. Instead, they need to learn as they go. In addition, the leadership progression for students can be steep. Students who take on leadership roles often do so after a semester or less of volunteer experience.

To support this rapid development, student movements need to provide training so that activists can develop necessary skills, ranging from event planning to public speaking. Training can be provided in many forms, including workshops, webinars, and conferences, and needs to be repeated often to accommodate the constant influx of new volunteers.

In addition to one-off trainings, movements need to provide the most talented students with long-term leadership opportunities that maximize their potential. For example, students in CfH's Campus Hunger Project Cohort program participate in an annual in-person gathering and monthly virtual trainings and receive individualized attention from program staff throughout the year. Programs like this help to develop the experienced leaders necessary for a successful movement.

The larger anti-poverty movement has numerous leadership development programs that can serve as models. Oxfam's youth engagement program runs the Oxfam CHANGE Initiative, which trains 50 students each year to organize on campus to end global poverty. These students attend an intensive week of training in the summer and get regular access to campaign materials and advice from Oxfam staff.[27]

An effective movement also needs to provide student activists who have cut their teeth on campus with ways to transition to the larger activist community after graduation. For example, the Emerson National Hunger Fellows Program at the Congressional Hunger Center gives recent graduates an intensive one-year crash course in social change. For the first half of the year, fellows are placed with a local community organization that provides direct services to people experiencing hunger. Fellows then spend the remainder of the year placed with national organizations working on hunger policy.[28]

These programs provide young activists with the essential elements for leadership development, including in-depth training, mentorship, networking, and hands-on experience. As the movement grows and more students become involved, groups will need to prioritize providing both entry-level trainings for new participants and in-depth leadership programs for the most talented students.

Provide Professional Support

Very few campus movements have been able to sustain themselves without the support of full-time professional staff. Student leaders turn over frequently as they graduate, transfer, study abroad, or leave school for other reasons. Having professional staff to support their efforts allows programs to experience continuity and growth, even as students come and go. Professional staff also provide access to networks and resources that student groups would find difficult to access otherwise. Staff can facilitate trainings, mentor emerging and established student leaders, and assist with difficult tactics that students might struggle with on their own.

For instance, the LGBTQ (lesbian, gay, bisexual, transgender, and queer) movement has numerous organizations with national staff who support student-led campus groups, most notably Campus Pride. Campus Pride was founded in 2001 to provide resources for LGBTQ organizations on campus.[29] Its national staff provides student activists with online guides and webinars, organizes a summer Camp Pride leadership academy, conducts academic research projects on LGBTQ issues, tours campuses with its Train the Trainer workshop series, manages a speakers' bureau, runs a Greek outreach program to support LGBTQ students in fraternities and sororities, and liaises with other organizations in the LGBTQ community. Its programs provide students with the professional support, leadership opportunities, and expertise to make the most of their efforts.

In addition to the staff employed by nonprofit organizations, student activists can also benefit from the support of campus administrators who work in student activities, civic engagement, and service learning. Due to their direct availability to students and knowledge of campus programs, administrators can provide day-to-day guidance to students in ways that professional staff from national organizations usually cannot. For example, professional staff have proven essential to the success of women's centers on campus. Women's centers, which were first launched in the 1960s and 1970s and are now commonplace, provide students with safe spaces, resources, and networks for activism, leadership development, and career-building opportunities. The advisors who staff these centers provide indispensable mentorship and support for feminist activism on campus.[30]

Shape Public Policy

The movement to end campus food insecurity began with programs like food pantries to address students' immediate needs and awareness campaigns to inform people about the problem. To tackle the root causes of hunger, students need to supplement educational campaigns and service projects with advocacy programs designed to change institutional, state, and federal policies. Doing so will not always be simple, but advocacy is vital to the long-term success of this movement.

Movement organizations can promote advocacy by providing students with policy analysis and support to help them engage effectively in tactics like writing op-eds for local and national media, sending letters and making phone calls to legislators, and holding lobby meetings. Students can be effective messengers by putting a personal face on the issue for policymakers, but their impact can be maximized with support from experts on navigating the policy process.

Local and regional advocacy programs like 1vyG can also be powerful forces for change. 1vyG is a network of first-generation low-income college students at Ivy League schools who are working to dismantle the financial, social, and academic barriers they face on campus. The 1vyG network has been successful in convincing institutions like Brown University and the University of Pennsylvania to waive application fees without requiring students to detail family financial hardships. Nearly 600 students gathered at the group's annual conference in 2018 to learn and share strategies for changing institutional policies. Notably, approximately 100 administrators also attended to discuss how to better support these students.[31]

The student hunger strike at Morehouse College and Spelman College is another powerful demonstration of student-led advocacy. Students at the colleges went on a hunger strike in November 2017 to protest campus policies that prevented students from donating their excess meal points to students in need. The strike was successful and ended when the administrations at both colleges committed to working with Aramark, their meal service provider, to establish a meal swipe donation program and to donate 14,000 meals per year for students in need.[32]

Students can also join together to create their own advocacy programs at the state or national level. For example, students have led the charge in Washington, DC, to protect and expand funding for federal financial aid programs such as the Pell Grant. Organizations such as the US Student Association and the US Public Interest Research Group have coordinated these efforts by providing students with the tools to influence Congress. Both groups employ professional staff in DC who lobby Congress on a consistent basis on students' behalf, organize lobby days where students meet with Congress members themselves, provide students with up-to-the-minute legislative updates, offer analysis on bills and amendments as they develop, testify at hearings, help students plan call-in days and petition drives, and coordinate with other DC policy groups. In recent years, their efforts have helped students win increases in the size of the maximum Pell Grant and fight back increases in student loan interest rates.

The campus food insecurity movement should create similar programs at the state and federal level to advocate for policies that would alleviate student hunger, such as increasing funding for work-study programs, expanding student eligibility for SNAP benefits, and streamlining the financial aid application process.

Movements Need Money

All of these resources require funding. It takes money to pay for staff, training materials, marketing, education, and the many other direct and indirect costs of running large programs. There are several different sources for funding large campus movements, including private donors, charitable foundations, and fundraising drives.

The university itself can be a source of funding for some activities, particularly at the local level. Campus-based organizations that operate with a chapter model often recommend that students register their chapters as student government–recognized clubs in order to have access to funding through student activities fees.

Corporate sponsorships are also a prospective funding source for some groups. For example, the 1vyG network enlisted elite firms like Bain Capital, McKinsey & Company, and Goldman Sachs to sponsor their annual student conference.[33] Given the increasing number of businesses that publicly champion social responsibility, there should be ongoing potential for investments from the business community.

For the movement to grow, students and professionals will need to work together to identify foundations and private donors who can provide the scale of funding necessary for large national programs. This high-level donor outreach will often fall to professional staff, given the skill and time required to develop donor relationships. However, students will play a vital role in these efforts by sharing their personal stories and experiences as a powerful way to demonstrate the importance and impact of their work.

Conclusion

There is reason to be excited about the potential for student activists to have a real impact on the issue of campus food insecurity. If organizations continue to pursue the recommendations described above, then students and allies will build a powerful movement and create a campus environment where all students have the support necessary to focus on their education rather than meeting their basic human needs.

Notes

1. James Dubick, Brandon Mathews, and Clare Cady, *Hunger on Campus: The Challenge of Food Insecurity for College Students* (Boston: National Student Campaign Against Hunger and Homelessness, 2016), https://studentsagainsthunger.org/hunger-on-campus/.

2. Robert Cohen, *When the Old Left Was Young: Student Radicals and America's First Mass Student Movement, 1929–1941* (New York: Oxford University Press, 1993), 188–93.

3. Maurine Hoffman Beasley, Holly Cowan Shulman, and Henry R. Beasley, eds., *The Eleanor Roosevelt Encyclopedia* (Westport, CT: Greenwood, 2001), 16–19.

4. W. J. Rorabaugh, *Berkeley at War: The 1960s* (New York: Oxford University Press, 1989), 47.

5. Clayborne Carson, *In Struggle: SNCC and the Black Awakening of the 1960s* (Cambridge, MA: Harvard University Press, 1981), 19.

6. Carson, *In Struggle*, 111–12.

7. Richard Knight, ed., *Sanctions, Disinvestment, and U.S. Corporations in South Africa* (Trenton, NJ: Africa World Press, 1990), 68–69.

8. "How Students Helped End Apartheid," University of California, http://www.universityofcalifornia.edu/news/how-students-helped-end-apartheid.

9. Kim Hopper, *Reckoning with Homelessness* (Ithaca, NY: Cornell University Press, 2014), 179–80.

10. Jerome P. Baggett, *Habitat for Humanity: Building Private Homes, Building Public Religion* (Philadelphia: Temple University Press, 2001), 71.

11. "Hands Across America," USA for Africa, http://usaforafrica.org/about-us/hands-across-america/.

12. Maureen E. Kenny et al., eds., *Learning to Serve: Promoting Civil Society through Service Learning* (Boston, MA: Kluwer Academic, 2012), 19–23.

13. Shelley H. Billig and Alan S. Waterman, eds., *Studying Service-Learning: Innovations in Education Research Methodology* (New York: Routledge, 2003), 1.

14. "History," Campus Compact, http://compact.org/who-we-are/history/.

15. Peter Dreier, "The Campus Anti-sweatshop Movement," *American Prospect*, Sept.–Oct. 1999; Jess Walsh, "Living Wage Campaigns Storm the Ivory Tower: Low Wage Workers on Campus," *New Labor Forum* 6 (2000): 80–89.

16. Sara Goldrick-Rab, *Paying the Price: College Costs, Financial Aid, and the Betrayal of the American Dream* (Chicago: University of Chicago Press, 2016), 1–22.

17. "Mission & History," Challah for Hunger, http://challahforhunger.org/mission-and-history/.

18. "Our Mission," National Student Campaign Against Hunger and Homelessness, http://studentsagainsthunger.org/about/.

19. Talia Berday-Sacks, Arielle Pearlman, and Carly Zimmerman, *The Campus Hunger Project Year 1 Report*, https://drive.google.com/file/d/0B6ZcCmdOHPn3X0xwLUM1clpxVzg/view.

20. "Crew Youth Collaborative," Enlight Foundation, http://enlightcollaborative.org/crew-youth-collaborative/.

21. "Learn about Know Your IX," Know Your IX, http://www.knowyourix.org/about/.

22. Nick Wing, "The March for Our Lives Was Inclusive. Here's How to Make Sure Its Agenda Is, Too," *Huffington Post*, Mar. 29, 2018, http://www.huffingtonpost.com/entry/march-for-our-lives-inclusive_us_5abbf6c9e4b04a59a3140efc.

23. Margaret Talbot, "The Extraordinary Inclusiveness of the March for Our Lives," *New Yorker*, Mar. 24, 2018, http://www.newyorker.com/news/news-desk/the-extraordinary-inclusiveness-of-the-march-for-our-lives.

24. "Youth at the People's Climate March," People's Climate March, https://peoplesclimate.org/.

25. "Dance Marathon," Children's Miracle Network Hospitals, http://dancemarathon.childrensmiraclenetworkhospitals.org.

26. "Meet IFYC," Interfaith Youth Core, http://www.ifyc.org/about.

27. "Frequently Asked Questions for CHANGE Leader Applicants," Oxfam America, http://www.oxfamamerica.org/take-action/volunteer/campus/change-initiative/change-faqs/.

28. "Emerson National Hunger Fellows Program: How It Works," Congressional Hunger Center, http://www.hungercenter.org/fellowships/emerson/how/.

29. "About Campus Pride," Campus Pride, http://www.campuspride.org/about/.

30. Susan B. Marine, Gina Helfrich, and Liam Randhawa, "Gender-Inclusive Practices in Campus Women's and Gender Centers: Benefits, Challenges, and Future Prospects," *NASPA Journal about Women in Higher Education* 10, no. 1 (2017): 45–63.

31. Valerie Strauss, "Low-Income, First-Generation Students Have—Finally—Established a Beachhead at Ivy League Schools. Now the Real

Work Starts," *Washington Post*, Mar. 13, 2018, http://www.washingtonpost
.com/news/answer-sheet/wp/2018/03/13/low-income-first-generation
-students-have-finally-established-a-beachhead-at-ivy-league-schools-now
-the-real-work-starts/.

32. "Morehouse, Spelman Students Hunger Strike Ends in Free Meals on
Campus," *TheGrio*, Nov. 11, 2017, http://thegrio.com/2017/11/11/morehouse
-spelman-students-hunger-strike-ends-free-meals-campus/.

33. "Partners," EdMobilizer, http://www.edmobilizer.org/partners-1/.

Student Action and Nonprofit Partnership

The Swipe Out Hunger Story

RACHEL SUMEKH

Editors' Prologue. Partnerships are part of many strategies addressing food insecurity among college students. There is tremendous power in collaboration and collective action. This chapter is a personal account of how forging internal and external partnerships can lead to creative programs that serve to address student food insecurity. One partnership between students at the University of California, Los Angeles, and their campus dining services eventually grew into a nonprofit organization that now partners with colleges and universities across the country to establish meal share programs.

About the Author. Rachel Sumekh is the founder and CEO of Swipe Out Hunger. The organization is a leading nonprofit in addressing hunger among college students by allowing students to donate their extra meal points to peers. Her work has been recognized by the Obama White House and the *New York Times*, and she was included on *Forbes*'s 30 Under 30 list in 2017.

When it comes to addressing student hunger, we must not be content with simply giving people food and treating them as though they cannot be part of the solution. Instead, we need to take it a step further by empowering others to create systems that become a part of the effort to support students' basic needs. Since 2010, Swipe Out Hunger has partnered with colleges and universities to end hunger, focusing not just on giving member schools a program but also on teaching them to develop and grow it over time. The way Swipe Out Hunger does this is through the Swipe Drive, which allows students with extra funds on their student meal plans to donate to their peers facing food insecurity on campus. Through the work of teaching colleges how to build their own Swipe Out Hunger program, the organization has learned ways to build strong campus partnerships, identifying key challenges and ways to address them.

This chapter focuses on the role colleges and universities play as partners in responding to campus food insecurity through the development of Swipe Out Hunger programs, sharing how the program gives students the tools they need to act and teaches colleges and universities how to address hunger on their campuses. This chapter will also touch on how Swipe Out Hunger seeks to transform the higher education food service industry into an equitable environment through policy and private partnerships.

UCLA—the Founding Story

I cofounded the first-ever Swipe Out Hunger program in 2010 as a 19-year-old undergraduate at the University of California, Los Angeles (UCLA). At the time, the movement to end student hunger was still developing and in need of new and innovative ways to address the issue of food insecurity on campuses. I felt frustrated by the number of unused meal swipes that I and my friends had left on our meal plans at the end of each semester, wondering why these swipes went unused while there were people in our community who did not have enough to eat. I decided to do something about it, bringing together groups of friends to enter the dining hall and purchase as many boxes of food with their extra points as they could carry. We then hand-distributed the meals to community members who needed them.

The responses from recipients of the food were positive. After hearing that the food came from students at UCLA, a recipient responded, "I had no idea you students gave a damn about me or knew I existed." That interaction made the group realize that an organized plan or program could have a lasting impact, helping members of the community feel seen and supported. After four days, the group of students had grown, and we had purchased and donated almost 300 boxed meals. I and the other leaders of the project set up a table outside of the dining hall where any student with extra meal points could "swipe" a box of food to be delivered to the community. We felt empowered and excited. The response had grown from one person's idea, to an action by a small group, to a community of people building a movement.

As the program grew and became more visible, I and my team were met with resistance from the university. On the fifth day of our tabling effort, a dining hall manager came over to investigate what we were doing. He slammed his hand on a box of food we had collected, saying, "This program is not happening on my campus. Stop immediately." For us 18- and 19-year-olds, the confrontation was jarring and presented a disappointing roadblock. We packed up the table and the boxes we had already collected, but we resolved not to retreat in response to this objection. Instead, we pledged to find a way for the program to continue. We decided to develop a plan to recruit dining services' support and form a partnership.

My team and I strategized ways to foster a positive relationship with dining services in order to continue the program we had named Swipes for the Homeless. We worked with the student newspaper to write an article about our work and what had happened, and members of student government reached out in response, offering to lend resources and their support to the effort. This partnership with the student body government played a critical role for Swipes for the Homeless because our team did not understand campus politics and how to work within the university system. Our partners within student government were well versed in how the campus worked and held a positive relationship with campus administration. My team and I worked with student government leaders to develop a game plan to reapproach dining services and see what could be done to keep the program going.

The Swipes for the Homeless team and student government met with dining and housing administrators about restarting the program. We knew that the conversation would be challenging. When meal swipes go unused, the funds are not returned to the student, but are instead kept by dining services. Getting permission to reopen the program meant persuading the university to give away tens of thousands of dollars in retail meal credit. At the start of the talks, the team was told that there was no viable way for the campus to support the program from a financial or logistical standpoint. The meetings were initially tense, but the Swipes for the Homeless team stayed committed to the end goal, worked to develop an understanding of what everyone wanted and needed, and formed a compromise that would work for everyone. After several months of negotiations, we reached an agreement with dining services, evolving from a program focused on the donation of prepared food to allowing students with extra meal credits the opportunity to donate them electronically at the end of each term. This was a much more effective and efficient way to collect donated swipes, and it could be done on a much larger scale. This new model addressed concerns around food safety and predictability, as dining services needed to be able to account for donated meals each semester.

In the new program model, donated funds were taken from students' meal accounts and placed into a newly named Swipe Out Hunger fund. At the start of the program, the recipient of the funds evolved each term. Swipe Out Hunger first donated to local food banks and soup kitchens in the community. One quarter later, the team had met a student who was launching an on-campus pantry to serve students and formed a partnership. We saw this as a great opportunity to support another student-led initiative by donating to the campus pantry. In partnering, Swipe Out Hunger provided the campus pantry with a consistent, reliable, and customized source of food. Some semesters we collected far more meal swipes than the pantry had space, so they continued to give the surplus to other organizations.

In 2011, my team and I were invited to meet with the UCLA Economic Crisis Response Team, a group created as a response to the recession. We learned that this team was offering supportive resources to students, including meal swipes that were purchased from dining services at retail price. The Swipe Out Hunger team saw this as an amazing opportunity to maximize our impact on campus. We rerouted the funds we were giving to off-campus organizations and invested them in what was named the Bruin Meal Voucher Program, or Bruin MVP.

As of the publication of this book, the Swipe Out Hunger program continues to support the UCLA campus pantry and issue meal credits directly to the accounts of students on campus. Since the founding of Swipe Out Hunger, new data have been collected to demonstrate the prevalence of food insecurity among UCLA students. In 2017, a campus study found that one in four students experienced consistent food insecurity at UCLA.[1] In response, the campus continued its support of the Swipe Out Hunger program, as well as providing paid staff for the food pantry and stabilizing its funding. The administration also offers a program called "Adulting 101," a pop-up resource fair including county social workers, financial aid staff, and other supportive resources to address students' basic needs beyond academics.

Success beyond UCLA

Swipe Out Hunger has expanded its work in addressing food insecurity among students, partnering with colleges and universities to help them develop their own meal swipe donation programs. After the program at UCLA gained visibility, students at the University of Southern California reached out, asking how they too could get their campus to allow the donation of extra meal credits. Our work continued to grow by engaging students one campus at a time. What started as a small project grew into a national network, taking the Swipe Out Hunger program to scale. By March 2012, I and the members of my team, who were at the time college seniors, were recognized by President Barack Obama for our outstanding work. The next part of this chapter shares how Swipe Out Hunger grew from a grassroots group of friends with an idea to a national program that has donated 1.6 million meals to students experiencing food insecurity. The Swipe Out Hunger team believes that the continued expansion and evolution of Swipe Out Hunger can be attributed to three key strategies.

Key Strategy 1

As an external nonprofit organization, Swipe Out Hunger builds campus capacity by providing important and valuable counsel to colleges and universities. The Swipe Out Hunger team trains campus leaders on how to develop meal donation programs on campus and consults with them during the process. From deciding who should be part of the conversation to determining how to finance the program and identify students facing food insecurity, Swipe Out Hunger provides colleges and universities with resources and support. Following the successful establishment of a chapter, the organization offers customized materials to help each chapter market its program in an effective way, ensuring that students know about the program and feel comfortable accessing it. Swipe Out Hunger has grown in its ability to help campus administrators quickly identify many of the potential challenges they could face when implementing this type of new initiative on campus and to offer proactive solutions in response. At the core of Swipe Out Hunger's national growth is clearly articulating its value to campuses as an external consultant and backing up its claims with useful tools such as case studies, trainings, and connections to similarly minded campuses.

These are what most attract campus leaders to a partnership with Swipe Out Hunger.

Key Strategy 2

Swipe Out Hunger seeks to empower local leaders rather than run individual campus programs. This has several advantages as well as challenges. Having started the program as students, the Swipe Out Hunger team saw the power of campus stakeholders to move the work forward from inside their own systems. This approach was inspired by the book *The Starfish and the Spider*. The book encourages companies to build *starfishes*, which are decentralized and can have arms cut off and still live and grow, as opposed to *spiders*, where each leg can only exist if still attached to the central core. The book uses the metaphor of the bodies of starfish and spiders to illustrate the value of parts that can operate independently from the whole.[2] The Swipe Out Hunger team built an organizational model where each of their member "arms" was just as strong and empowered as the core.

Swipe Out Hunger seeks to both attract and train leaders like Jordan, a third-year college student in New Jersey. When he reached out with interest in our program, asking when we could send a Swipe Out Hunger representative to his campus, the reply was, "Congratulations, you're the new rep." Jordan stepped up, and with the support of the Swipe Out Hunger team, he was able to start a program that is still running successfully today. Taking this approach empowers local individuals to lead the work and make it their own. This strategy leads to three key outcomes: engaged and invested campus leaders, a highly scalable and flexible program, and an agile and flexible headquarter team that can focus on training and consulting for programs, rather than building them. This outcome is how Swipe Out Hunger has been able to support programs on 75 campuses across 28 states with only four full-time staff.

Key Strategy 3

Swipe Out Hunger is adaptive to an evolving environment and the stakeholders it serves. From the beginning, Swipe Out Hunger has received five to six new campus inquiries each month. Initially, all of the interest came from students. Thus, Swipe Out Hunger developed student-specific trainings and resources to prepare students for the process of working with administrators. The materials provided what was needed to launch a program, including data on student hunger and guidance on how to connect with the right campus stakeholders. Over time, partner demographics changed, and by 2017 half of the inbound interest came from campus administrators, rather than students. Because administrators require different support from that of students, the Swipe Out Hunger team evolved in their approach to develop best practices, case studies, and other tools to train and support new partners. Swipe Out Hunger now shares ideas and models from across the country, helping administrators successfully launch their programs. My team and I believe that remaining agile is key to providing the best support to our partners—no matter who they are.

Swipe Out Hunger credits its success to learning from the mistakes and challenges of the past and seeking solutions so that they are not replicated in the future. Swipe Out Hunger also seeks to learn from the mistakes of other nonprofit organizations, identifying and addressing the challenges many nonprofits face, including management of overhead, growing capacity while scaling, and finding a way to maintain a strong organizational culture. The Swipe Out Hunger team seeks to create a model that avoids these challenges by considering and addressing them before they become issues. Today, Swipe Out Hunger studies the partnerships that universities create with for-profit corporations as models, asking questions about what makes these partnerships work and what drives them. For example, "What leads a university to pay millions of dollars for things like software platforms or dining services?" or "Why do campuses choose one dining services company and not another?" As a service provider, the Swipe Out Hunger team also seeks to help members clearly communicate their program's value and design a program in which colleges and universities are willing to invest.

A Series of Case Studies on Swipe Out Hunger
Developing a Growing Partnership—University of California, Santa Barbara

Shannon was a freshman when she emailed Swipe Out Hunger regarding starting a Swipe Out Hunger program at her campus, University of California, Santa Barbara (UCSB). From the first call in 2013, it was clear that Shannon had passion and an entrepreneurial spirit but very little familiarity with the UCSB campus and its bureaucracies. The Swipe Out Hunger team advised Shannon to pitch her idea to someone in her student government and have them join her team so that she could benefit from their expertise in navigating campus politics and systems. Shannon reached out to Ali, a junior who was running as a candidate for student body president. As a person immersed in campus politics, Ali quickly became passionate about Swipe Out Hunger's mission and added it to her campaign platform.

The Swipe Out Hunger team trained Shannon and Ali on how to prepare a proposal and helped them identify the key campus administrators from whom they needed support. The team also shared a long list of reasons why the campus might reject the program, enabling Shannon and Ali to develop responses to potential objections in advance of a meeting. Within two months of Shannon's initial email, Swipe Out Hunger had trained Shannon and Ali, who in turn felt confident and ready to meet with administrators. The student leaders were prepared to address campus administration's concerns during their first conversation, avoiding being told to come back with answers. The Swipe Out Hunger team knows that bureaucratic systems like colleges and universities tend to push things off, and we see our role as advocates and mentors helping students overcome that challenge through preparation and planning.

Shannon and Ali had a very positive and successful meeting. Their dining administration was sympathetic to the issue and agreed to allow Swipe Out Hunger to operate, provided that the team did not collect more than 75 meals per quarter. On a campus with 20,000 undergraduate students, this was a woefully tiny number, but rather than lashing out, the two students thanked the administrators for agreeing to the program and asked whether they could report back on the progress. They anticipated that their fellow students would quickly outpace that cap.

Shannon and Ali assembled a team of volunteers, and within 30 minutes of setting up a table they had collected their 75-meal allotment for the quarter. They returned to the dining administrators and shared this success, along with an article in the campus newspaper that demonstrated the general enthusiasm for the program among students across campus. They used these data to ask for an increased cap, and it was raised to 250 meals per quarter. Every academic term for the next year, the students continued to treat dining services as a true partner, keeping them updated and asking for an increase to the cap. Within one year, the students had been granted a 3,000-meal cap, which they still easily filled. In addition to developing this strong partnership with administration, the Swipe Out Hunger team at UCSB worked with their campus pantry, student government, student housing, Greek life, and neighboring homeless shelter to grow the meal voucher program and increase its impact. As of 2019, through stronger collaboration between the Swipe Out Hunger team at UCSB and the campus pantry leaders, they were successfully able to obtain a 6,000-meal cap per year.

Fighting Hunger at a Private Liberal Arts College—Ithaca College

In January 2017, a freshman named Unagh reached out to the Swipe Out Hunger team with the goal of setting up a program to help classmates who faced food insecurity. Unagh had heard that in the past the Sodexo food services partner on campus had allowed students to donate funds from their meal plans to support an off-campus charitable cause. This gave the Swipe Out Hunger team hope that it would be feasible to develop a partnership targeting student hunger. Over the course of the next year, Unagh made connections with various stakeholders across campus, including the coordinators of the mobile food pantry, service-learning staff, ICare case management staff, religious institutions on campus, and student organizations focused on hunger. Unagh sought to educate these different parties on the issue of college student hunger and generate interest in starting a meal donation program on campus.

In February 2018, the Swipe Out Hunger team worked with Unagh to finalize a program proposal for the executive director of auxiliary services. They compiled data from the Swipe Out Hunger programs at other Sodexo campuses, including demographics and retention data and the number of students who used the pantry at Ithaca College. Next, Unagh identified a staff member in financial services who was able and willing to take on the role of distributing swipes to students. The Swipe Out Hunger team worked with Unagh to file a formal proposal that included the necessary logistics for starting a Swipe Out Hunger program at Ithaca and the benefits of having such a program. Finally, in April 2018, Unagh and a few other student leaders on her team participated in a Swipe Tank competition, where they practiced presenting their pitch to a panel of Swipe Out Hunger alumni judges, getting feedback to incorporate into their real presentation. By July 2018, Unagh's team had presented their case and received approval from Sodexo to start a pilot Swipe Out Hunger program in the fall of 2018. The Swipe Out Hunger team spent the rest of the summer supporting Unagh in putting together a plan to market the donation drive and perform outreach targeting the students who needed the meals.

The first Swipe Drive took place August 29–September 19, 2018. A total of 949 students signed up to donate one of their guest meal swipes to help stock an emergency meal bank, which was housed in the Financial Services Office. By November 2018, half of those meals had been given to students across campus, and the Swipe Out Hunger student group at Ithaca College grew to 13 team members. Their team hosted a series of Hunger and Homelessness Awareness events, and the president recognized Unagh for her leadership at the Ithaca College Community Honors awards ceremony. The partners at Ithaca have since gone on to introduce the Swipe Out Hunger team to other universities in the region so that they can learn about how to start their own meal donation programs.

Working with Community Colleges—Santa Monica College

I would not have made it through the year if I did not have the meal vouchers and the food pantry program.

—First-generation college student at Santa Monica College

The Swipe Out Hunger model works well on the campuses of four-year institutions because they all have dining halls and meal plans with swipes to donate. However, in 2016 the Swipe Out Hunger team began receiving interest from community colleges, which presented a creative opportunity for Swipe Out Hunger. While serving a new sector, including campuses that do not have meal plans, could be challenging, the Swipe Out Hunger team recognized the stance it needed to take as an organization committed to ending student hunger. According to national data, community colleges have the highest share of food-insecure students, so the team wanted to quell doubts that its program could serve these campuses.[3] The Swipe Out Hunger team deliberately expanded its work to community colleges because we believed that if we were to be ultimately successful as an organization addressing student hunger, the program should apply to *all* students.

Developing a model for community colleges began with a listening tour. The Swipe Out Hunger leadership met with and learned from community college administrators and students at the six community colleges in the city of Los Angeles. At the core, we kept our philosophy of leveraging existing resources on campus and in the community. What we found, however, was that in many cases the programs and services the Swipe Out Hunger team relied on as foundations for their programs at four-year institutions did not exist at community colleges. We eventually started an experimental partnership with Santa Monica Community College (SMC) to help develop a series of programs designed to ensure that students' basic food needs were met. Together with SMC administrators and students from SMC's student government, we supported the creation of a new and creative way to provide students with meals: the Free Lunch Voucher program.

The Free Lunch Voucher is a free lunch ticket worth five dollars. Each food retailer on campus agreed that if a student were to bring them this voucher, they would provide the student with a whole, healthy meal—often a simplified version of what the retailer already sold. The program's initial funding came from a student fee referendum where a dollar from student fees was taken and added to the fund. In its first year, the program could support 1,400 students with these lunch tickets. Following the Free Lunch Voucher program's success, the dean of student life at SMC removed the onus of paying for the program from students by asking the college professors to donate $19.42 from each paycheck toward the initiative. This was a positive and well-branded campaign that gained tremendous support among faculty and raised $45,000 in its first year.

Addressing the Challenges

Through strong partnerships with colleges and universities, Swipe Out Hunger ensures that they have the knowledge and capacity to move their programs past challenges, such as student volunteer turnover or lack of funding, to sustainability. While there are many nonprofits dedicated to getting students ready for college, the focus of Swipe Out Hunger is to get the colleges ready for their students—particularly, students who come from backgrounds where they are more likely to face food insecurity. The Swipe Out Hunger team draws from the observations and lessons gleaned to ensure that new programs are well prepared for the students coming to their campus and set up to successfully serve them. This section outlines some common challenges and how Swipe Out Hunger helps their partners overcome them.

Making Room for a New Program

Colleges and universities have large and complex bureaucracies that maintain their operations. When presenting a new basic needs program, the Swipe Out Hunger team often encounters reluctance to introducing something new. There is a fear that adding a new program can impact the success of other programs or systems—such as existing dining services on campus. In working with colleges and universities, the Swipe Out Hunger team helps address these concerns in advance, often introducing a smaller pilot program to demonstrate how it could work without disrupting important systems and services. Once the pilot is implemented and assessed, many of the concerns of the university are addressed and the campus can move forward knowing what it would take to scale the program and how much they can afford to invest. For example, many campuses are concerned that managing the program will drain the time of their dining staff. Upon launching a pilot, campuses recognize that the time commitment consists of (1) moving funds from student accounts to the Swipe Out

Hunger fund and (2) quarterly meetings—both of which are usually deemed reasonable if their Swipe Drives are limited to three a year.

Financing a Meal Share Program

The biggest question the Swipe Out Hunger team gets is how to finance a meal share program. In response, they offer different models and provide guidance on which approach is best for the campus. The most basic model is to allow students to share their extra meal swipes and cap it at the number of meals the school can sustain. Additionally, campus departments that have flexible budgets to create new programs, like the Office of the Dean of Student Life, can set up a fund to start Swipe Out Hunger to serve their students. Many campuses fund pilot programs (and even ongoing programs) by leveraging student fees. Others utilize state and federal programs, such as Cooperating Agencies Foster Youth Educational Support and other targeted funding. This is often a feasible approach for community colleges. Finally, there are several local philanthropic foundations funding campus anti-hunger programs, such as the Leichtag Foundation in San Diego and the Good People Fund in New York City. In some cases, Swipe Out Hunger can introduce foundations to colleges in their geographic focus area.

The Desire to Be Unique

For many schools, the *U.S. News and World Report*'s annual campus ranking is very important. The competitive nature of a ranking system drives campuses to invest in innovative and impressive programs. This is one reason why some campuses choose to develop a Swipe Out Hunger program. Additionally, some campuses wish to leverage their program to garner press interest or engage in fundraising. This can be particularly exciting to alumni who may have experienced hunger on campus and wish to support a program they would have benefitted from in the past.

Their Students Need It

Some college administrators, faculty, or students understand the urgency of serving students who are facing food insecurity. This could be because they have measured food insecurity on campus or because they are familiar with students in need. Recognizing food insecurity as a threat to student success and college completion drives many colleges and universities to start a Swipe Out Hunger program on campus.

As an organization, Swipe Out Hunger must gauge these priorities and help the campus meet their goals. For instance, one Ivy League campus partner has focused on the role student leaders play in the program since student civic engagement is core to their culture. Thus, Swipe Out Hunger ensures that student leaders remain at the center of the conversation and receive adequate support. The Swipe Out Hunger team knows that if those students are strong, so will be the university's investment in the program.

Maintaining the Relationship

Partnership goes both ways. The Swipe Out Hunger team knows that it is important to come to the table with a clear understanding of the university's needs and interests. We know we need to be clear in communicating how the partnership would benefit the campus and its students before expecting willingness from the university to share data, resources, or information. The university should seek to be a good partner as well. One of the important lessons learned is that a positive partnership is based on clear communication and good relationship building.

University staff, as with nonprofit staff, wear many hats and often have limited capacity. The Swipe Out Hunger team works to create a partnership where our emails and phone calls are prioritized by campus staff. Everyone on the Swipe Out Hunger team is trained in the basics of community organizing, which teaches ways to authentically share values and goals and solicit the same from others. By finding shared values, the relationship can be sustained beyond transactional tasks. Swipe Out Hunger utilizes a customer relationship management technology platform so that its staff can record detailed notes. By referencing these details in future communications, university partners are reminded that Swipe Out Hunger is invested in them. This relationship continues to deepen if Swipe Out Hunger can help the campus point person take ownership of the program. The organization supports and engenders this buy-in to cultivate personal investment. This ensures that partners will remain creative and determined as they seek to support and grow the program.

Swipe Out Hunger's best partners go above and beyond in ways that do not strain their capacity, and the team ensures that campuses have what they need to make it easy to do so. Swipe Out Hunger is generous in sending campuses stickers, T-shirts, posters, pins, and other branded materials. While these are a minor cost to Swipe Out Hunger, they are meaningful swag items that help partners feel like an important part of the Swipe Out Hunger community. It also helps advertise the program. Swipe Out Hunger provides partners the opportunity to broadcast their work to the public, as well as higher education leaders, through newsletters, publications, newspapers, and social media. Each university partner is added to the Swipe Out Hunger website, and a new webpage is created for them with details about their program and other resources to address food insecurity on campus. Swipe Out Hunger invites campus leaders to generate blog posts to highlight their campus's programing and collects and shares program data twice a year through reports and public appreciation posts.

Program Evaluation

The Swipe Out Hunger team knows the importance of collecting data and assessing the impact of a program to further justify its importance and secure resources to sustain it. In 2018, we conducted a nationwide survey of the program. Campus leaders in charge of the meal donation program distributed the survey to student beneficiaries. Swipe Out Hunger offered a $10 incentive to every student who responded and contracted a professional firm to assist with the process. The survey was conducted on nine university campuses and received 843 responses from student beneficiaries.

The findings were encouraging. After receiving swipes, students reported a 48 percent decrease in the need to skip meals or eat less than they should because they could not afford food, a 49 percent decrease in their reliance on a diet of processed food, a 46 percent decrease in their worries that food would run out before getting money to buy more, and a 57 percent decrease in their tendency to lose weight because they did not have enough money to afford food. In addition, students shared the following remarks:

I've become more resilient to stressful situations now that I am eating regularly.

—Student at a private liberal arts college in Minnesota

The free dining hall pass has made me realize that UC Irvine really cares about its students and will not let me fail by providing help with food. It made me feel like I am important on this campus.

—Student at University of California, Irvine

I have met a couple of friends in the dining halls and have even ran into others that share my situation. We now support each other.

—Student at California State Polytechnic University, Pomona

This program is very supportive and makes me feel more secure about my financial situation and my overall health, this program lets me know that Cal Poly cares about its students.

—Another student at California State Polytechnic University, Pomona

With dining passes I don't have to resort to cheap unhealthy food which in turn helps me feel better and better about myself.

—First-generation student at Rutgers University

Sharing these data with campuses enlightens the administration of the prevalence of this issue on their campuses. To effect change for each of its campus partners, the Swipe Out Hunger team developed tailored presentations and reports with campus-specific data alongside national numbers. Campus contacts then held meetings with campus administration to present the data and slideshow. Andrea Gutierrez, the basic needs coordinator at University of California, Irvine, said that their campus leadership was "impressed by the presentation," and before her team could even make the request, their dining services team increased the number of available meals by 500 for the year.

Basic Needs and Legislation

Public higher education has gone from being largely state and federally funded to relying heavily on student tuition. There is an urgent need for local, state, and national representatives to prioritize higher education to ease the incredible financial burden associated with college today. As the movement to address student food insecurity evolves, there have been a handful of state and federal representatives who have taken bold action. Swipe Out Hunger has been able to provide support for this work.

In March 2017, I received a call from Assemblywoman Monique Limón's office. Limón had just been elected to the California legislature following her tenure as a student support administrator at UCSB. Her legislative director told me they had seen the impact of Swipe Out Hunger at UCSB and were interested in learning how the program could scale to every college in California. The Swipe Out Hunger team educated the representative's staff on the varying needs across California's higher education systems, emphasizing that the meal donation program alone would not suffice. When the representative asked what would, I drafted potential proposals based on providing funding to campuses to develop approaches tailored to their needs and the needs of their students. Assemblywoman Limón's office approved of the suggestions, and Swipe Out Hunger became an official coauthor, working to push the bill forward. Swipe Out Hunger gathered endorsement signatures and a Senate cosponsor. In April 2017, I traveled to Sacramento to testify on behalf of the bill. At the end of the day, the bill successfully made it out of committee. In May 2017, Governor Jerry Brown signed the Hunger Free Campus Act into law, adding $7.5 million in incentive funds.

After the bill's passage, I asked the representative why she reached out to Swipe Out Hunger rather than other leaders in higher education or anti-hunger. The representative told me that Swipe Out Hunger's "outsider affiliation" made it a perfect fit since the organization was independent, unfunded by any political movement, and unaffiliated with any agenda other than supporting college students. She saw the partnership with Swipe Out Hunger as a way to develop meaningful legislation while avoiding any appearance of bias, which hinders many political processes.

Swipe Out Hunger believes that policy responds to public and cultural shifts, rather than the opposite. Initially, Swipe Out Hunger was an innovation that was too disruptive and foreign to campuses. After the program started, the Swipe Out Hunger team witnessed a culture change as the program was adopted one campus at a time. Donating meal swipes became a more accepted practice in higher education. This gave Assemblywoman Limón and the state legislature enough confidence to move the program and bill forward.

In the year following the passing of the bill, many other legislators have proposed legislation to support basic needs work on campuses. Swipe Out Hunger does not support all proposed legislation, but instead works with lawmakers' staff to shape bills into what would actually work. In one instance, a lawmaker introduced a bill that would give scholarships to all low-income students to cover the cost of a meal plan on their campus. The bill would cost the state $500 million dollars. The Swipe Out Hunger team believed that the funds could be better spent focusing on solutions that result in upstream change. The appropriations committee agreed and did not approve the bill. Several months later, in May 2018, I testified again before lawmakers on the issue of student hunger. When asked what types of laws I would suggest for creating upstream change, I suggested that they should address the contracts campuses are signing, with both food providers and technology providers, ensuring that students' interests are met before businesses' interests.

Conclusion

Clarity of mission is central for any nonprofit or community organization. The Swipe Out Hunger mission has evolved to become more refined. When it began in 2010, the team was driven by the desire to use meal points for good in the community around UCLA. From 2010 to 2012, we homed in on testing how viable and sustainable it was to build partnerships with other universities. From 2013 to 2015, after some universities signed on to create programs, we sought to leverage dining dollars and partner relationships for the most good—investing wholly in the issue of college student hunger. From 2015 to 2017, an increase in understanding of the issue on campuses meant that the Swipe Out Hunger team did not have to spend as much time and resources explaining and convincing universities of the problem. Instead, we could go straight into developing the program. We developed a less flexible and more turnkey approach to consulting and campus support.

Today, the Swipe Out Hunger team continues to strive to be better partners for colleges and universities. We seek to partner with other nonprofits, such as local pantries and national organizations like Feeding America, to play a pivotal role in addressing student hunger. We know that informing partners makes them more successful in serving students. Other health care–focused groups and nonprofits, such as the American Heart Association, are emphasizing a closer association between food and health, leading to potential partnerships in the future. Additionally, a core group of organizations, including Swipe Out Hunger, the College and University Food Bank Alliance, Challah for Hunger, and others, are working more closely together on a shared plan of action.

The business sector has also turned its attention to the issue of college student hunger. While attending a conference in Chicago in 2014, I heard the vice president of a major campus food provider state that Swipe Out Hunger's model was neither sustainable nor scalable. At the writing of this book, that food provider and another major one are interested in meeting to discuss a partnership to support students. As the Swipe Out Hunger team considers the potential impact the private sector could have on the issue, we feel hopeful—especially considering the growth of our program over the past five years. We also believe that administrators can incentivize good business practices by encouraging campuses to stipulate that companies include basic needs programs like Swipe Out Hunger in contracts. Swipe Out Hunger believes that corporate social responsibility has become more about making the business look good and less about making the public good a part of its mission, and it seeks to bring these big players in the food industry to the table.

Finally, the Swipe Out Hunger team believes that students and university leaders are the future of the work and is investing now more than ever in those who run its programs by bringing them together for leadership trainings. By connecting with alumni mentors and engaging its board of young professionals, Swipe Out Hunger keeps those who have already graduated engaged and as part of leadership. The team is also working with students willing to speak publicly about the issue in front of groups and the media, seeking to center the focus on student voices and stories.

Notes

1. University of California Global Food Initiative, "Global Food Initiative: Food and Housing Security at the University of California," *University of California Office of the President*, Dec. 2017, https://www.ucop.edu/global -food-initiative/_files/food-housing-security.pdf.

2. Ori Brafman and and Rod A. Beckstrom, *The Starfish and the Spider: The Unstoppable Power of Leaderless Organizations* (New York: Portfolio, 2006).

3. Sara Goldrick-Rab et al., *College and University Basic Needs Insecurity: A National #RealCollege Survey Report*, Apr. 2019, https://hope4college.com /college-and-university-basic-needs-insecurity-a-national-realcollege -survey-report/.

[6]

The Trampoline of Public Benefits

Using Existing Resources to Fight Food Insecurity

SARAH CRAWFORD AND NICOLE HINDES

Editors' Prologue. Beyond partnerships between food pantry programs and local food banks, some colleges are turning to other external agencies and programs to bring existing resources onto campus for their students. Public benefits, including the Supplemental Nutrition Assistance Program (SNAP), can bring much-needed monies for students to pay for food and other basic necessities. The challenge is that even when students meet the stringent qualifications for public assistance programs, they may not enroll because the application process is complicated and often conflicts with students' class and work schedules. This chapter discusses two different on-campus models for supporting students as they pursue public benefits, while also offering additional wraparound services that can help meet students' basic needs.

About the Authors. Sarah Crawford serves as national education director for Single Stop, a national nonprofit that partners with colleges and nonprofit organizations to connect low-income individuals to resources that help them achieve financial self-sufficiency. Sarah began her career in case management for the federal government, supporting individuals in connecting to benefits and resources. She has worked for nearly two decades in both government and nonprofits in the areas of higher education, poverty alleviation, policy development, and health and human services. She is a graduate of North Carolina (NC) State University and serves on the NC State University School of Public and International Affairs Board.

Nicole Hindes, a first-generation college student, graduated from Indiana University with a master's in education and has spent over a decade working directly with underresourced, low-income college students. She has led the Human Services Resource Center at Oregon State University since early 2016, successfully integrating the data-informed best practices she learned in the nonprofit sphere. When she is not doing economic justice work, she enjoys developing her meditation practice or finding immersive peace in a beautiful landscape.

The evidence is clear: students are dropping and stopping out of college because their basic needs are not being met.[1] Too many students have to decide between books, groceries, tuition, and a safe place to sleep. Financial aid is not enough to cover the real cost of college, and we are losing students, some before they even enter. While there has been considerable focus on these issues in the past five years, the conversation started earlier than that.

The first decade of the twenty-first century was marked by an increased focus on postsecondary access and completion by higher education leaders and politicians alike. President Barack Obama, for example, announced plans to close gaps in college access and completion for low-income and minority students and called for an additional 5 million college graduates by 2020. To reach this goal, institutions could not simply rely on increasing enrollment; colleges and states also needed to align resources to support degree attainment.[2] In the years since, states, higher education institutions, and individual practitioners have taken significant steps to promote student success through resource coordination. In this chapter, we focus on the work of two organizations that independently emerged in the early 2000s and seek to improve educational outcomes by fighting poverty.

The Human Services Resource Center (HSRC) is a homegrown initiative by Oregon State University (OSU) students, and Single Stop is a national anti-poverty nonprofit organization that partners with community colleges and other organizations that serve low-income families across the nation. Though the organizations are distinct from one another, they share a common strategy: connect students to the social safety net or similar campus programs so that they can leverage existing resources to push toward a degree while making ends meet. Moreover, both organizations utilize a one-stop approach that serves as a central on-campus hub where students can go to find a supportive staff member who can help them troubleshoot and create a plan to meet their basic material and educational needs.

The Beginnings

Both organizations have learned, over the course of their work, that connecting students to benefits and resources is not easy. The web of social services is complex, and so both organizations needed to start small and leverage existing resources and partnerships, while building their programs for greater impact.

At OSU, students saw firsthand what their peers were experiencing as the price of tuition and living costs increased. Their roommates were dropping out of college and leaving vacant rooms with costly lease obligations, classmates were skipping meals, and friends were sleeping in the library or couch surfing. The students took action before administrators had a chance. In 2000, student government leaders created the first service, an insurance premium subsidy called the Student Health Insurance Subsidy. The program was designed to alleviate some of the financial burden placed on international students, who were required to have health insurance (something not yet required for all domestic students). A few years later, in 2005, students started to directly address the problem of hunger and food insecurity on campus. The Student Committee on Hunger and Poverty launched the Escape Hunger Project, which relied on volunteers to cook lunch that was then provided for free to as many as 500 students each week. In the following years, students replaced the Escape Hunger Project with the Mealbux program, which provides students with funds to access existing campus food services, and also added a campus food pantry.

In 2008, two OSU students formalized efforts to help their peers make ends meet with a proposal for the HSRC—a place on campus modeled after Human Services offices in most communities. The students put forth a vision for a one-stop center where those experiencing homelessness, food insecurity, and poverty could receive the wraparound support that they needed. That is, students could complete Supplemental Nutrition Assistance Program (SNAP) applications with trained support, get basic groceries from a food pantry, take a shower, do laundry, and get additional services. The students even pitched the idea of emergency shelter beds within the facility. Though the students did not have a lot of data to make their case, they had confidence that what they were seeing in the early years of the Great Recession was not the sole source of their friends' economic challenges. They knew somehow that these challenges would continue to exist over a decade later. They were right.

Single Stop began in the broader community, rather than in an institution of higher education, but with similar goals to the HSRC. Single Stop builds on a simple idea: fight poverty by providing financially vulnerable households with coordinated access to public safety net programs, postsecondary education, jobs, and financial self-sufficiency. Michael Weinstein, one of the founders of Single Stop, started the anti-poverty program in the basement of a church in a poor neighborhood in West Philadelphia and brought it to New York City in 1990. In 2002, just two years after OSU students started taking action, Weinstein took the idea to the Robin Hood Foundation, an anti-poverty charity operating in New York City, which proceeded to create Single Stop sites through partnerships with community-based organizations in many of New York's poorest neighborhoods.

In 2007, Elisabeth Mason, Herb Sturz, and Mr. Weinstein—with generous help from the Atlantic Philanthropies—turned Single Stop into a separate 501(c)(3) nonprofit organization. What had started out in a cramped basement in Philadelphia soon took on national proportions. Today, Single Stop offers a one-stop off-ramp out of poverty by supporting families in meeting their basic needs. Throughout its history, Single Stop has focused on essentials: sites connect visitors first and foremost to food stamps, local food pantries, housing programs, and jobs.

Single Stop employs a partnership model in which it provides sites with computer software with which to screen individuals for eligibility for public benefits, a case management tool, expertise in benefits and wraparound services (i.e., tax, legal, and financial counseling), and tools for collecting and analyzing data. Partners implement the Single Stop program, providing space and staff and welcoming walk-in visitors to one-on-one counseling in friendly, neighborhood settings. Partner sites also refer visitors to other community-based organizations, providing a local support network. The early impacts of this network approach were clear. In its first two years of establishing itself as a stand-alone nonprofit organization, Single Stop served over 170,000 individuals, connecting them to $389 million in benefits and resources. Single Stop was beginning to gain traction in New York City, and other organizations were taking notice.

Expanding Services

By combining social and education services with Single Stop's technology, programmatic training, data and evaluation tools, and consulting expertise, Single Stop aims to create organizational shifts in the way colleges approach student retention, with the goal of improving outcomes for both students and schools. Though Single Stop began as an anti-poverty effort in community-based organizations, it quickly became apparent to the organization that there was tremendous need among college students. In 2009, the same year that the food pantry at OSU started serving students, leadership from Kingsborough Community College in New York City approached

Single Stop after learning that their students were seeking human services resources, including food supports, off campus, in the broader community. Kingsborough Community College's question was simple: can we help meet the basic needs of our students by putting a Single Stop program on our campus? The answer was yes!

In 2009 Single Stop partnered with Kingsborough Community College, and soon after it partnered with five additional community colleges in the City University of New York (CUNY) system. In 2010, more than 5,700 CUNY student households received more than $8.3 million in public benefits such as SNAP, WIC (Special Supplemental Nutrition Program for Women, Infants, and Children), and health insurance and in local aid resources such as food pantries and housing supports. The benefits that students were connected to at the highest rate were for food supports in the form of SNAP and WIC, which suggests significant need in this area. Though students often seek help as a result of hunger, once they are connected to Single Stop, they learn about eligibility for and receive help in accessing other public benefits (e.g., tax credits, Low-Income Heating and Energy Assistance Program) and additional on- and off-campus resources (e.g., clothing closets) that can supplement their income and help meet their basic needs.

Today, Single Stop has expanded its college initiative to more than 33 sites across 10 states. Over the years, Single Stop has refined its model in higher education and provided evidence that meeting the basic needs of students through benefits access can change students' trajectory by giving them an opportunity to become more successful in school.[3] Single Stop's work in higher education is based on a theory of change that relies on embedding services and institutionalizing the Single Stop model on college campuses so that students can access resources and services that they need to stay in school.[4]

OSU students, on the other hand, did not rely on computer software or statistics to implement their programming. They watched their peers struggling in school and directed student fees toward programs and initiatives that brought more resources to under-served students. Due to healthy enrollments, the student government, Associated Students of Oregon State University (ASOSU), under which the HSRC was developed, experienced budget growth and created a team of staff who worked on basic needs issues. Student staff provided oversight for the insurance subsidy, the Mealbux campus food assistance program, and an on-campus emergency housing program where students could stay in one of two designated residence hall rooms. Initially, a graduate student oversaw programming, and then the first professional staff member, Clare Cady, was hired. As both need and support for these programs increased, funding grew as well. When the campus sought a bond measure to build a collection of smaller buildings on campus, a funding source was identified to support the renovation of a small former cooperative residence hall with the explicit purpose of housing the HSRC.

As the design and construction processes progressed, the HSRC became autonomous from ASOSU, with its own budget and oversight. Professional staff turned over, and Nicole Hindes was hired in 2016 as the program moved into a new permanent home. The new space includes a large, professional pantry; a commercial-grade kitchen; a shower; plenty of office space; a laundry room; and social gathering places where students can relax, build community, or take a nap.

Today, the HSRC operates from a perspective of abundance—the idea that we have the resources to meet students' needs and do not need to operate from a mind-set of scarcity. Most HSRC programs have been borne from students' ideas, and most labor and effort are a result of student employees and volunteers. An advisory board consisting of students, staff, and community members informs annual budget conversations, as well as programming and service delivery. Major projects are run by students, with oversight and guidance from professional and graduate student staff. Services are offered with minimal gatekeeping—each program has its own requirements, and most are designed to be as simple and stream-lined as possible.

Single Stop in Practice

Similar to HSRC, Single Stop is embedded on college campuses, and while HSRC utilizes human power to run all of its programs, Single Stop uses technology to support its work. When a college or university first partners with Single Stop, its national staff work with the college to conduct an analysis that includes an overview of student need on campus and on-campus resources available to students. This work culminates in developing goals for Single Stop on that particular campus, including key metrics related to the number of students served and the amount of benefits and resources to which students are connected. The college identifies staff to oversee the Single Stop office, and that individual (or individuals) is responsible for supporting students, outreaching to students, and developing the on- and off-campus partner network for students. The college may hire new staff or reallocate existing staff to support the work of the Single Stop office, including screening students for benefits and connecting them to resources using the Single Stop technology. The college staff for Single Stop offices also serve as case managers, following up with students who complete the screening to ensure that they received the identified services and inquire about their well-being to see whether they need additional resources.

The Single Stop approach to partnership, which is dependent on the college context, can take many forms and can work in various geographies with different-sized student populations. Similar to the ways in which HSRC expanded the types of services available for students, Single Stop college partners work to meet the needs of their student body. In addition to core services (e.g., benefit screenings and case management, free tax preparation, and financial and/ or legal counseling), college partners often also include campus services, such as emergency grant funding and food pantries, as part of their Single Stop office. We provide some examples below.

At Nash Community College, located in rural Rocky Mount, North Carolina, with a student population of approximately 5,000, the college did not create a new office for Single Stop or immediately hire new staff, as some college partners have done. Instead, the college embedded Single Stop in its existing Student Wellness Center and placed the director of student wellness over the program acting as the Single Stop director on campus. Nash also worked immediately to incorporate existing campus-developed resources into its Single Stop program. This includes their Blue Love Fund, an emergency aid program that supports students with basic needs insecurities through items such as grocery gift cards in a more immediate way.

Delgado Community College (DCC), located in New Orleans and with a student population of 19,000, created a new Single Stop office and a new director position, which has been the more common way to bring Single Stop to a campus. While not all campuses have the luxury of having multiple staff for their Single Stop office, DCC also hired an assistant director and utilizes interns to support their work. DCC created a Single Stop office on their main campus, City Park, and DCC Single Stop staff also travel to their branch campuses weekly to ensure that they are serving all DCC students. Delgado's Single Stop office is specifically addressing food insecurity through the establishment of a campus food pantry, the Care Corner, which staff created after seeing so many students who were not able to say, with confidence, where their next meal would come from. The food pantry is colocated with the Single Stop office on campus, so that students can get the supports that they need in a one-stop shop.

At the four-year institutions that have partnered with Single Stop, the approaches are varied to meet the needs of the institutions. At Johnson C. Smith and Winston-Salem State Universities in North Carolina, staff who were already supporting students—but without the combination of technology and social services—were reallocated to be the Single Stop directors. At the University of Massachusetts Boston and John Jay College, staff were newly hired to run the Single Stop office, but it was colocated with existing student services.

Food Security Evolutions at Oregon State University

For more than a decade, OSU has been implementing multiple food security solutions. No one program is a panacea. A student parent with two custodial children has different sources of food insecurity than the student in the residence hall who finds her dining plan empty with two weeks remaining in the term—a food pantry often works great for the parent, but not for the student living in a traditional dorm room. These challenges present in varied ways for food-insecure students—sometimes a lack of knowledge or time, and sometimes insufficient skills or tools. However, the root cause of food insecurity is financial pressure; insufficient financial aid (or other economic resources) puts pressure on how much time a student needs to spend working and how much time they have left to study. Many HSRC students experience both food and housing insecurity concurrently. Thus, food security solutions at the HSRC include literally handing students food as well as developing programs that alleviate the underlying financial pressures that can cause food insecurity.

HSRC Food Pantry

The HSRC Food Pantry, formerly called the OSU Emergency Food Pantry, is part of a local food bank network. The HSRC uses a modest account with the OSU Foundation to cover the costs associated with receiving food from the regional food bank—some of which have no cost because they are distributed as part of the US Department of Agriculture's (USDA) commodity goods program. Because of this partnership, for which the center receives pallets of food for pennies on the dollar, the resource is also available to eligible community members or staff. To receive food from the HSRC Food Pantry, individuals sign a form, sharing their name and address and attesting that they meet the income eligibility requirements. No identification, proof of address, or proof of income is needed.

Each person who visits the pantry has the opportunity to receive food for three to five days, including an allotment of vegetables, grains, proteins, and dairy. The HSRC has shopping-style distribution days about four times per month, during which clients are matched with a volunteer who helps them go through the options and choose their own food items. Outside of these designated days and times, clients can visit the pantry and ask for an emergency box of food to be prepared for them. Clients will receive the same quantity of food but cannot shop in the same way. In the 2017–18 school year, the HSRC distributed an average of 18 pounds' worth of food per individual, which includes about 5 pounds of fresh produce. The cost of supporting this resource is about $2.26 per visitor per visit. The campus food pantry is one of the most popular and cost-effective services at the center, with an average meal cost of about 14 cents, before labor or facility charges. In contrast, the program's Mealbux food voucher program, described below, costs about $7 per meal.

HSRC Food Assistance Programs

When the aforementioned Escape Hunger Project became difficult to run owing to significant volunteer staffing coordination and financial costs, student leaders replaced it with the Mealbux fund in 2009. The goal of providing students with healthy and nutritious meals did not change, but the new voucher program model cut down on the significant administrative strain that was associated with the Escape Hunger Project. The new vision is to provide funds directly on a student's ID card so that they can purchase a meal anywhere on campus at a time that is convenient for them.

Initially, Mealbux awards were worth $250 per 11-week term, or about $23 per week, enough to cover the average cost of three to five meals at campus restaurants and cafes. In developing the program criteria and formula for Mealbux awards, student leaders met with financial aid officials and designed a numbers-based application that would take into account a student's financial situation (e.g., tuition costs, financial aid award) and resources (e.g., contributions from family, employment income) to create an assessment of unmet need. The student leaders wanted to create their own measure of eligibility and resource distribution, rather than rely on the Free Application for Federal Student Aid (FAFSA), since international and undocumented students are usually ineligible for federal financial aid. Since demand for the resource outpaced funding, restrictions were put in place: applicants had to complete a paper application within the first week of each term and attach documentation of their financial aid award or income statements. Early awards were first come, first served, and when students had complaints about fairness and accessibility, staff tried a random awarding process where not all applicants received funds. Finally, staff settled on a distributive model—those in the applicant pool determined to have need would be awarded funds, split with all other eligible applicants in the pool. The more students who applied, the less everyone got, but everyone who applied with need got some Mealbux award amount. Over time, some nuance was added such that those with higher financial need received $20–$40 more than those with medium or low need, and an appeal process worked to catch those who may not fit the standard evaluation. Initially the program was run with an Excel spreadsheet, and it was eventually upgraded to an Access database. Over the years the database became cumbersome and slow, making it challenging to summarize data. As these initial challenges were addressed, new ones appeared. For example, some students applied for the program without realizing that Mealbux was meant to address food insecurity, and staff had to spend hours doing data entry for hundreds of applications. The process had become too confusing and too challenging to assess. A new system was needed.

In fall 2017, the HSRC launched the Food Assistance Application, an online application used to award Mealbux and connect students to other resources. Due to the online format, students can complete the application anytime, day or night, during the first week of the term. Instead of opaque, numbers-based calculations, students are asked directly about their experiences with food insecurity using both the USDA's Food Security assessment questions and a series of other internally developed questions that staff suspect might be more applicable to college students.[5] Students are also asked about their experiences with generational or situational poverty, about their housing security, and a selection of other questions that automatically feed into email-based interventions for other support. The application screens for SNAP eligibility, likely reasons why a student might want to revise their FAFSA, and likely need for a dozen overlapping services (e.g., childcare subsidy offered by another campus office). The application takes an average of 20 minutes to complete—though the questions are accompanied by simple check boxes. No complex calculations are needed, and very little information is asked for that a student would not know off the top of their head. Thus, students complete the Food Assistance Application both to assess their food insecurity and as a screener to identify ways in which the HSRC can connect students to other sources of support. If a student indicates high or pressing need, a staff member may reach out directly to offer support or a more high-touch level of assistance, in addition to food subsidy funds. The data gathered from this application help the office provide data-informed program changes and report, with more accuracy, to stakeholders about the challenges that students are experiencing as tuition and costs of living rise while financial aid stagnates. The online application resulted in a roughly 25 percent increase in applicants, but the data collected also led directly to a significant increase in funding during a recent budget negotiation. Today, the application awards nearly $220,000 in annual food assistance at OSU.[6]

HSRC SNAP Access

Data from the first year of the Food Assistance Application clearly illustrated the need for greater attention to SNAP efforts on campus. Over 500 unique students indicated that they were likely eligible for

SNAP but reported not receiving the assistance. Over a year, this is nearly $1 million of noninstitutional aid these students could be collectively receiving. However, the SNAP application is challenging. Questions on the application are difficult to understand, student eligibility is confusing, and state workers sometimes make errors that further complicate eligible students' likelihood of approval. Historically, the HSRC has invited Department of Human Services staff on-site during the academic year to help students complete SNAP applications. Inconsistencies, confusion about timing, and dynamic student schedules have prevented this from working well. Recent attempts to email students to encourage them to complete applications have had very low success rates. In January 2018, the HSRC held a "One Snap, Get SNAP" large enrollment event so that students could meet with an eligibility worker and start an application that day. Multiple computers were available, multiple trained staff provided application assistance, and over 50 students participated. It was a successful first year, but there is more work to be done connecting students to this helpful resource.

In fall 2018, the HSRC launched a SNAP Ambassador program to continue to address this challenge. The center staff recruited work-study students who became SNAP Ambassadors, and they completed a short training covering the basics of completing a SNAP application, student eligibility clarifications, and destigmatizing information about food insecurity. SNAP Ambassadors wear an "Ask me about SNAP!" button and talk with their friends and classmates about SNAP eligibility and basic information. Most work-study students, after completing the training, realized that they are eligible for SNAP as well (because of their work-study status), and hopefully they have received sufficient training to complete an application and advocate for themselves in the eligibility screening process. If students need to requalify for SNAP in future terms by working additional hours in their work-study employment, they can table on campus about SNAP and HSRC resources or perform other outreach to destigmatize food insecurity. The idea is to use the network to both reduce food insecurity stigma and help students meet a basic and easy eligibility requirement for student SNAP participation.

HSRC Textbook and Housing Programs

Food and textbooks often compete for students' last dollars since tuition and rent are typically paid first. In winter 2018, an HSRC student explained, "Textbook and lecture materials are very expensive, and I have to cut my meals and eat once a day because I need to save money to buy lecture materials. Sometimes I have to lie to my friends whenever they asked me to go for a lunch by saying that I've already cooked at home." The Textbook Lending Program (TLP) helps students avoid food insecurity in two ways: (1) saving them money on books that can now go toward groceries, and (2) helping students learn about HSRC food security programs. Functionally, the TLP provides a core outreach function for the center. From a student perspective, going to a strange, new office across campus and asking for groceries or food support can be a high barrier to overcome, especially if the student is nervous about his need or the likelihood that he will find appropriate resources. However, most students are frustrated by the high costs of course materials, and so the TLP provides an opportunity for students to save a few dollars on textbooks by visiting the HSRC, where they can also meet friendly staff and learn about food security resources. The TLP provides term-long loans for textbooks and other course materials, but each book includes a sticker inside that also explains to students that they can come back to the HSRC for assistance with food or housing security needs.

Textbook and course material loans are distributed, generally, on a first-come, first-served basis. The first week of each term is for priority access students, including those who are Pell Grant eligible, participate in the campus federal TRiO-funded programs, have a SNAP benefits card, are a veteran or have a military ID, or are former foster youth. Students who are low-income or otherwise financially stressed (e.g., undocumented students) can work with professional staff to be included in the priority access group on a case-by-case basis. After the first week of the term, all OSU students can check out any remaining textbooks. Materials are organized and loaned using the same databases as the campus library, which means that anyone with an internet connection can look to see whether their textbook is available via the HSRC.

The HSRC has offered this program for two academic years, and both the textbook library and its use are growing quickly. Initial funding came from a small grant from the OSU Foundation Women's Giving Circle ($10,000) and program matching funds (another $10,000). Annually, the HSRC spends $20,000 in program funds to grow the library. The initial purchases included course materials from the 30 courses taken most frequently by Pell Grant–eligible students. Future purchases have and will continue to be made by students requesting their book via a survey each term in which they list what books and course materials they need. The HSRC textbook library has grown much faster than anticipated; more than half of the books currently in the collection came from donations from students, staff, or faculty. During the first year of the program, the HSRC loaned 99 books to students; in the second year of the program, the HSRC loaned 1,140 books. A total of 1,077 books are currently in the library and available for checkout.

Additionally, the HSRC provides housing supports since worrying about food usually becomes secondary to worrying about having a roof over one's head. The HSRC Emergency Housing resource has also been a benchmark of success in supporting students' basic needs. This partnership with the campus housing office, University Housing and Dining Services, holds two residence hall spaces for HSRC use throughout the academic year. Students who are homeless or at imminent risk of homelessness can, following an intake at the HSRC, stay in one of the rooms at no cost for up to 28 days while they find a more permanent solution. This resource is very useful for students who fit a traditional college student experience, whereas those with more complex living situations (e.g., they have dependents or pets or are not able to live in a community setting) often cannot use this resource.

Additional HSRC Food Security Initiatives

In addition to the food security and closely related textbook and housing programs described above, the HSRC continues to innovate and develop new initiatives to fight hunger on campus. Below, we briefly describe some of the latest efforts.

Twitter.—Another successful food security intervention has been the simple creation of a Twitter account, @eatfreeOSU, that posts all events on campus that have free food available for students. Within the first academic year, nearly 900 students, staff, parents, and community members started following the account. HSRC student staff search for campus events that have free food, take note of flyers advertising programs, and accept submissions from event planners. Tweets include not only details about the free food and logistics but also language that encourages students to get involved, build leadership skills, or learn something new. Occasionally after an event ends, students or staff across campus will tweet at the account offering students the opportunity to show up and eat leftovers before catering comes to clean up. In the first year, the account posted about 230 events, an average of seven events per week, where students could eat for free.

Full Plate Funds.—Full Plate Funds are similar to Mealbux, but they are only for students with a dining plan who have run out of dining dollars. Unlike Mealbux, Full Plate Funds can only be used in dining halls overseen by the campus housing and dining department. Also, the program is supported by student donations, similar to the swipe programs discussed in chapter 5, whereas Mealbux is supported by student fees.

Facilities.—HSRC staff buy food in bulk and repackage the food in smaller portions for household distribution via the food pantry, thanks to the commercial-grade kitchen facilities. When not in use by the program, the HSRC kitchen is available to any OSU community member to use to prepare a meal. A community fridge is also available for students sleeping in vehicles or without adequate refrigeration facilities who need to keep their food cold. Future plans to fully license the kitchen will allow the space to be used to prepare on-site-catered meals to students, should the program develop that or a similar concept for program growth. HSRC's large space also works well for student clubs that might want to hold an end-of-year potluck, furthering relationships across campus.

Forgot My Lunch.—A "forgot my lunch!" counter display provides basic ingredients so that any student across campus can stop by the HSRC and grab a lunch kit, can of soup, or snack so they do not have to spend money (that they do not have) to buy a meal on campus. Similarly, when someone cancels a catered lunch on campus at the last minute, the catering team often brings the food to the HSRC for distribution.

Cooking Classes.—Students are excited about cooking classes. Usually, 10–20 students come to learn from volunteers, staff, or community members about anything from stepping up a ramen noodle dish to cooking basics, like making rice or bread. In January 2018, a "Seed to Supper" series, in partnership with OSU Extension Services, had about 15 students attending a six-week series where they learned to grow their own food for supper.

Production Garden.—An on-site production garden, managed in partnership with a student sustainability group, provides locally grown fresh produce such as herbs, greens, vegetables, and fruit. Harvested food is used during instructional programs or distributed via the food pantry.

Cookbook Library.—A library provides term-long loans of basic and specialized cookbooks, including multiple copies of Leanne Brown's *Good and Cheap: Eat Well on $4/Day* (roughly a SNAP budget).[7] It also includes several books about meal prepping and cultural food recipe books, as well as some that examine the culture and tradition of food as a concept and some that look at classism and poverty through a food lens.

Small Appliance Library.—HSRC has future plans for a small appliance library where students will be able to check out an instant pot, food dehydrator, food processor, and other items that can be expensive up-front purchases but can help keep costs down over the long term.

The HSRC food security programs are more successful and numerous than other HSRC programs for multiple reasons. First, as the program has built them out, it is evident that they are serving different populations of students, who have different sources of food insecurity. Many international students appreciate the food pantry, through which they can receive enough food for their entire family. Students in highly rigorous academic programs who are too busy studying to work sufficient hours often appreciate the flexibility of the Food Assistance Application and the funds they award. Those who might not have the skills to cook for themselves on a budget are drawn to the cooking classes and workshops. These programs are useful for students who live off campus, whereas the Full Plate Fund, for example, is designed to serve on-campus or traditional first-year students. Other programs try to meet students' financial challenges in other ways.

Impact

Since beginning its work as a stand-alone nonprofit in 2007, Single Stop and its partners, including community-based organizations, have connected 1.8 million households to more than $5.9 billion in benefits and resources. With specific regard to the work with college partners, more than 269,000 student households have been served and more than $548 million has been drawn down in benefits and resources for students. Data collected show that students who are eligible for public benefits receive $5,500 on average per year through connections made by the Single Stop office; this is nearly equivalent to the size of a federal Pell Grant. In the 13 years the HSRC has been providing food assistance funds (both Mealbux and Full Plate Funds), approximately 20,000 OSU students have received a total of $1.6 million. Campus dining staff believe that this estimate translates to approximately 250,000 meals.

Our work over the past two decades has taught us that hunger can first bring a student to the one-stop office, but students are often eligible for other benefits and services as well. According to Single Stop's data, the top three services provided to students are food pantry referrals, enrollment in food stamps, and food assistance (free meals). The total number of students supported in these three areas among Single Stop's college partners is 70,391, representing nearly 54 percent of the more than 130,000 students that have received any type of benefit enrollment. The HSRC also sees how students are often skilled at getting their needs met with multiple resources. Through the 2017–18 school year, 1,704 unique students used HSRC programs (not all programs track individualized data), participating in over 10,791 service points.

In 2018, nearly one-quarter of Single Stop students served were connected to multiple benefits. For example, the student may have received both SNAP and a tax credit. For example, Judy, attending community college part-time to become a nurse, was working three jobs to provide for her family.[8] She was struggling to pay her bills and keep up with her schoolwork when she visited the Single Stop office for help. Judy ended up being eligible for many benefits, with a combined value of $12,000 per year. Judy was able to quit not one but two of her jobs, allowing her to focus more of her time on school and graduate on time.

Understanding the role of multiple benefits is important. While we do not often think of some of these benefits, such as tax credits, as being ways to support students who are food insecure, if the student can be connected to a different benefit or credit that puts money in their pocket, many stressors can be alleviated, including food insecurity. The HSRC does similar work with the Textbook Lending Program, for example.

Single Stop has also been the subject of evaluations by RAND Corporation and Metis Associates. In these studies, researchers have sought to show the relationship between receiving Single Stop benefit screenings or other services and academic performance. These evaluations found that students who received Single Stop services were more likely to persist toward graduation than their peers who did not. Depending on the campus and how the program was implemented, the results ranged anywhere from 3 to 15 percentage points. Key implementation factors include oversight from top administrators, strong program staff, a collaborative approach, a strength-based perspective, and foresight into potential roadblocks. These results suggest that the integration of Single Stop services makes an impact for both students and their colleges.[9] The HSRC will be exploring some of these same questions in the coming years.

In addition, there are also countless personal stories of impact. Many students, as noted earlier, are facing hard decisions of whether to stay in school or get a second job in order to afford food. Colleges across the country have story after story of these types of cases, and Single Stop is no different. Helen from Charlotte, North Carolina, enrolled at Central Piedmont Community College (CPCC) and was on the brink of dropping out so that she could get a job. She was homeless, with a 2-year-old son. Like so many who face homelessness, she did not have enough food to eat herself and had barely enough for her child. She did not have consistent childcare for her son and did not have access to reliable transportation to get her back and forth to school. Helen found the Single Stop office at CPCC and told them she had a dream of graduating from college, but she was on the verge of having to give up on that dream. Through Single Stop, she was connected to the local food bank, food assistance, childcare, and transportation. She was also connected to local housing options. All of these benefits and resources worked together to meet the basic needs of her and her son. Helen stayed in school and completed her degree, putting her family on a path to economic stability and self-sufficiency.

Lessons Learned

The collective experiences of these programs show that multiple factors are necessary to help students meet their basic needs and address student food insecurity on college campuses. These lessons include having the right support from leadership and the right resources allocated, gaining an understanding of the complex world of benefits, and using data to inform program development and promote student success.

Campus Support and Partnerships

Regardless of who is accountable to supporting student food security, no one office or one person can do it alone. Partnerships and support—from senior leadership to students and staff with "boots on the ground"—are essential to program success. In the case of bringing the Single Stop program model to a campus, it is not simply about bringing another initiative on campus. Instead, it is about embedding and integrating the service on campus, which means that there needs to be a network of faculty, staff, and administrators that support and facilitate its success. At the HSRC, each initiative requires willing partners to collaborate, share in the labor, help promote programs, and problem-solve when things get challenging.

Thoughtful Staffing, in Both Approach and Structure

It is not uncommon for this work to start as a portion of a campus staff person's role, though a best practice includes at least one full-time professional person leading the program. Staff need to be skilled in relationship building, student outreach, and the development of faculty/staff and community partners. Specialized skills such as technological competency (important with Single Stop and use of web forms related to the software), case and project management, instructional skills, fundraising, and marketing can also go a long way. At the HSRC, the staff has learned that additional program growth and more students served means that additional full-time equivalents are needed to support facility and logistical needs.

Start Small and Be Strategic

Providing holistic supports and benefits access on campus can be complicated. Successful sites start small and are strategic about their rollout. One two-year college campus, for example, wanted every single person to walk away from a new Single Stop office with a positive experience, even if they were not eligible for benefits. Instead of opening up the office widely in the beginning, they took appointments and prescreened students. If students were not eligible for public benefits, then they were offered a grocery card or transportation card so that they received some assistance and left praising the program. In less than three years, that Single Stop site has connected 688 students to more than $4.3 million in benefits.

The HSRC also started small and strategically, adding new programs slowly. Providing this type of support to students is somewhat new in the United States, and it can take time to develop a comprehensive model. At OSU, each new program or initiative had to clear hurdles, both with buy-in and in terms of logistical supports. Adding programs slowly over the years has been a successful strategy that also lends itself well to sustainability over time. Each new program or initiative is best served by a standardized repeatable process that is recorded and has plans for training and integrating new project coordinators as student staff graduate and leave the university. Relying on a single person, who has not recorded the workflow or processes, is risky and often causes headaches later.

Data Collection

At the beginning of a new initiative, it is important to consider what types of data you will collect and how it will support and justify the costs of the program. Partner sites utilize the data and evaluation tools provided by Single Stop to report on the number of students served and the dollar amount of benefits provided to students. The HSRC shares its data similarly and also collects personal accounts of program impact, but sometimes campus leadership needs more information. In these cases, institutional research departments can be a resource to help conduct basic program evaluations that can provide evidence of the program's value to campus.

Data and evaluation can also be used to consider what growth or expanded services could look like, and a strategic plan can be invaluable when a major donor expresses interest in providing financial support. In addition, sites can use data to advocate for certain programs and services. For example, a student at James Sprunt Community College in Kenansville, North Carolina, did not have adequate transportation to and from school, and the county did not have a decent transportation system. As a result, he had been walking 11 miles, one way, to school, so he went to Single Stop to seek help. The college utilized data that Single Stop had collected about the number of students needing transportation to successfully advocate for new and elongated bus routes to serve their students.

The Future of This Work

Over the past decade, OSU—and the HSRC in particular—has taken a students-serving-students approach to addressing food insecurity and hunger. Most HSRC programs are the result of student ideas, and most of the labor to support these programs has been provided by student workers. The result is that students take real leadership and initiative in their work. Since its inception, student coordinators have overseen the food pantry, completing reporting requirements, managing inventory, and monitoring food safety with very little professional staff oversight. Similarly, students overseeing the Textbook Lending Program are using the back end of a rather complicated library database system (Alma) to run reports, enter materials, create staff users, and complete other complex functions. These students are receiving real-world, highly applicable skills that can contribute to their future professional success.

The limit of student employment, however, is successfully case-managing a student in financial crisis. When the HSRC was a new program and had fewer partnerships to manage—and a different facility—professional staff had more time to spend supporting students in crisis. As more administrative requirements were needed and program growth added complexity and new relationships to manage, the HSRC needed professional staff time set aside to case-manage and work closely with students in crisis. In summer 2018, the HSRC gained a second full-time professional, given the title of basic needs navigator, who provides the needed case management services to students; this person also builds and maintains relationships with landlords and community agencies to help students with pressing financial concerns.

Future growth at the HSRC will include a third full-time staff member who will support the food security efforts of the program and free up the director to build relationships with donors, support research, and develop more student-friendly affordable housing opportunities. The HSRC will also integrate more class identity–based conversations and dialogue into programming to build a better campus understanding of social justice frameworks around income inequality and socioeconomic status. Students also expect the HSRC to be a place where they can get skills-based workshops on topics like managing student loans and tips on purchasing a vehicle, budgeting, and meal planning. At the same time that HSRC staff are providing this content to the student body, they are also integrating opportunities to advocate at campus, local, and state levels for the funding and support needed to address the root causes of housing and food insecurity.

In the years since Single Stop began its college initiative in 2009, it has expanded to more than 33 sites across 10 states. As Single Stop looks ahead to the next decade, the organization is committed to the following three tenets:

1. *Supporting Existing Partners.*—Single Stop's strength is in its college partners. We have learned through the years that supporting existing partners really means the following: providing support and technical assistance on benefits screenings and the case management tool; training site staff on benefits eligibility, advocacy, and applications; consulting with sites on how to expand services on their campuses; and connecting partner sites with each other to gain perspective on best practices from other campuses.

2. *Expanding Services to Reach More Students.*—Single Stop is committed to providing services where requested and needed. As more and more colleges have expressed an interest in partnering with Single Stop, Single Stop has streamlined its work and is expanding into new states, with our sights on eventually expanding to all 50 states.

3. *Improving the Program Model.*—Single Stop is committed to taking what it has learned through the years and what it will continue to learn to improve the technology, consulting, training, and evaluation. This will better support partners in their work to improve student outcomes.

Single Stop also has an opportunity to shape and inform public policy by leveraging its national network to identify how access to resources can be more effectively streamlined and coordinated on the federal, state, and local levels. Single Stop is committed to promoting college affordability and works to advance the adoption of evidence-based strategies for college retention and completion so that all students may have the opportunity to succeed.

Conclusion

As we entered the 2010s, there was a distinct focus and agenda for improving college completion, which, in part, led to a growing body of research about why students are not completing college. Increasingly, college leadership and student support staff are beginning to understand, as well as witness, that nonacademic barriers like food insecurity are a significant obstacle to college success. The two programs presented in this chapter offer unique approaches to reach the same end goal of keeping more students in school. We believe that helping students access resources in the short term improves their chances of long-term success via postsecondary education.

Whereas Single Stop has thrived in a few key areas—utilizing technology, staff-led case management, and quantitative data collection—the HRSC has thrived in student leadership, integrating programs, and qualitative data collection. Single Stop's scaled technology solution would be even more impactful by learning from the HRSC's truly integrated student-led support model and incorporating that into the work. Conversely, Single Stop has created a robust case management model, led by staff, that could alleviate some of the growth stressors that the HRSC has experienced. While both models have proven successful, there is an opportunity for campus communities to leverage the strengths of both programs, drawing on the lessons learned over the past decade of doing this work, to create a sustainable program with maximum impact for students.

It is also important to consider the data in order to see not only the impact of these types of programs but also that systemic change can be informed and influenced in a way that makes it more likely that students will succeed. Arguably, the data and research indicate that hunger is a key issue facing college students. The data also point to the fact that supporting students who are food insecure can increase the chance that they will graduate.[10] While there are countless opportunities to impact campus-level policies with this information, there are also longer-term solutions that need to be made when it comes to state and federal policies that can be informed by the findings of these types of programs and other research.

Notes

1. For a review of the problem, please see chap. 1. "Stop out" refers to a pattern of enrollment where students leave college but return in subsequent semesters or years; it emphasizes the complex experiences of today's college students and is often used in contrast to simply "dropping out" and never returning to college.

2. Davis Jenkins and Thomas Bailey, "How Community Colleges Can Reach Obama's Goals," *Inside Higher Ed*, Oct. 13, 2009, https://www .insidehighered.com/views/2009/10/13/how-community-colleges-can -reach-obamas-goals.

3. Lindsay Daugherty, William R. Johnston, and Tiffany Tsai, *Connecting College Students to Alternative Sources of Support* (Santa Monica, CA: Rand Corporation, 2016), https://www.rand.org/pubs/research_reports/RR1740 .html; Jing Zhu, Michael Scuello, and Susanne Harnett, *Single Stop Impact and Implementation Report: Phase II Findings* (New York: Metis Associates, Jan. 2018), http://www.metisassociates.com/our_work/downloads/Metis _07-16_SingleStopReport.pdf.

4. Single Stop's theory of change is predicated on the following: (1) Poverty reduces millions of Americans' ability to participate and contribute in a vibrant economy. Postsecondary education is a powerful lever for low-income Americans to move out of poverty. (2) More than 40% of college students drop out, many as a result of financial barriers; Esmé Aston, "Why Students Drop Out of College, and How We Can Do Something about It," *Huffington Post*, Jan. 16, 2018, https://www.huffingtonpost.com/entry/why -most-students-drop-out-of-college-and-how-we-can_us _5a5d9f77e4b01ccdd48b5f46. (3) Many low-income college students and their families are eligible for, but do not claim, billions of dollars in existing benefits and services. If accessed, these resources could bridge the financial gap that prevents students from completing.

5. Other questions used by the HSRC Food Assistance Application to assess food insecurity with college students include the following: (1) How often do you skip meals to make your dining plan last longer? (2) Do you usually run out of dining plan dollars before the end of the term? (3) Do you seek out events and activities on campus that provide free food to save money? (4) Does your family help your budget go further by sharing groceries, prepared meals, or leftovers when you visit them? (5) Do you eat cheap, low-cost convenience meals to save money? (6) Do you eat cheap, low-cost convenience meals to avoid feeling hungry? (7) Have you used food pantries in the past 12 months to feed yourself or your family? (8) Do you avoid social activities with friends or classmates because you can't afford to

go out with them? (9) Do you feel pressure to hide how stressed you are about affording food from your family and those who care about you?

6. This total includes Mealbux and Full Plate Funds, discussed below.

7. Leanne Brown, *Good and Cheap: Eat Well on $4/Day* (New York: Workman, 2015), https://cookbooks.leannebrown.com/good-and-cheap.pdf.

8. All student names have been changed to protect their identity.

9. Daugherty, Johnston, and Tsai, *Connecting College Students*; Zhu, Scuello, and Harnett, *Single Stop Impact*.

10. Daugherty, Johnston, and Tsai, *Connecting College Students*; Zhu, Scuello, and Harnett, *Single Stop Impact*.

[7]

Transformational Change for Student Success

The California State University Basic Needs Initiative

DENISE WOODS-BEVLY AND SABRINA SANDERS

Editors' Prologue. This chapter demonstrates how an entire university system is working to promote food and other basic needs security so that students can reach their academic, career, and life goals. Grounded in a framework that includes five tenets for addressing basic needs in a higher education setting, the authors provide several university case studies to illustrate how they scale single-campus best practices system-wide. The chapter concludes with reflections and recommendations for a systems-level approach to fighting hunger on college campuses. The case study continues in the next chapter, written from the perspectives of faculty whose research spurred action to address food insecurity across California State University campuses.

About the Authors. Dr. Denise Woods-Bevly is a public health practitioner currently serving as the director of the Student Wellness and Basic Needs Initiative for the California State University, Office of the Chancellor. In this position, she provides system-wide leadership of programs and services that address student well-being across the 23 campuses, impacting roughly half a million students. Her work includes engaging various well-being constituents, encompassing student health services, student mental health and counseling services, and food and housing security.

A 20-year veteran of higher education, Dr. Sabrina Sanders currently serves as the director of the Student Affairs Projects & Initiatives for the California State University, Office of the Chancellor. Her focus has been on eliminating equity gaps and increasing completion rates to ensure that all students have access to the opportunities provided by a high-quality college degree. Follow her @SabrinaKSanders.

Chancellor's Message

Food and housing insecurity affects students at every college and university in the country. The California State University (CSU) and its sibling institutions across the state are no exception.

We know—through data and anecdotes—that when students are constantly worrying about their next meal or whether there will be a roof over their head that night, they have less time and mental energy for academic study and success.

While the challenges of ensuring basic needs are widespread across the country, the CSU stands as a trailblazer in research and action—leading efforts to better understand the issues and offer meaningful and sustainable solutions.

In 2015, I was inspired by the story of a student and the passion of a faculty member to commission a study of food and housing insecurity within the CSU. The initial goal was to take a snapshot of the needs of students on just a few CSU campuses. While we knew that the need was great, we did not know the full extent—or depth—of the crisis.

We soon learned—thanks to the initial research of Dr. Rashida Crutchfield and her team at CSU, Long Beach—that the crisis was widespread and persistent. Through similar studies by our sibling institutions, we also learned that the need was equally pervasive across all of higher education.

There was much to do, and we got right to work. As you will read in this chapter, the CSU community is turning knowledge into action.

Today, for students struggling with food insecurity, all 23 CSU campuses have a food pantry or food distribution program. More than half of our campuses offer meal-sharing and meal voucher programs.

For those students facing housing insecurity, more than two-thirds of our campuses offer emergency on-campus housing or vouchers for off-campus housing. All told, the CSU has supported thousands of students through these offerings.

We have made a lot of progress, but we are not done.

In the months and years to come, the CSU will further expand and strengthen its outreach to the most vulnerable students, connecting them with resources, counselors, advisors, and centers.

The CSU will also strengthen partnerships with the University of California and California Community Colleges; state, county and municipal governments; and philanthropic foundations to improve continuity of services and build holistic assistance for students and their families.

When the first phases of the CSU Basic Needs Initiative were launched, we declared that it is our responsibility—as educators and as Californians—to make certain that every student impacted by food and housing insecurity can receive the support they need to achieve their lifelong, dream-driven goals.

Today—through the dedication of thousands of CSU employees, students, alumni, and friends—we are breaking down silos, sharing critical data across campuses, and developing best practices that will make transformational impacts on basic needs research and action.

Today, we help every CSU student—regardless of circumstance or background—reach their dream-driven academic, career, and life goals.

Chancellor *Timothy P. White*
The California State University

Mission of Service

Education has a unique role as a gateway—or, in its absence, a barrier—to social mobility, economic prosperity, and civic responsibility.[1] The California State University (CSU) system was born of the idea that a quality comprehensive higher education should be accessible to all, serving students beyond the walls of the classroom. Persistent food and housing insecurity denies students access by creating barriers to academic participation and degree completion. These artificial barriers are contrary to the CSU's public purpose and mission. Therefore, the CSU has systemically engaged in the work of addressing student *basic needs.*

The CSU engagement in basic needs is a natural extension of its service model. The 23 CSU campuses are not just in the community; the expectation is that most draw the majority of their student population directly from surrounding communities. Campuses are hubs of social and educational partnerships to provide outreach and services. Faculty and students conduct directed research to address community challenges in community settings.

This idea of a community-focused state university was revolutionary when the California Master Plan for Higher Education was established in 1960.[2] Its importance centered on the principle that higher education would be available to all regardless of economic means. Many states and nations have since adopted elements of the California Master Plan, as competitiveness in the global knowledge economy has increasingly relied on a citizenry that continues its education past high school.

In serving California's communities, the CSU student population has grown to half a million students. This population is among the largest and most diverse in the country. More than half of the university's student population are people of color, and one-third are the first in their families to attend college. Rooted in its public mission, the CSU also serves an unprecedented number of low-income students. More than 221,000 CSU students rely on federal need-based Pell Grants.

With some 120,000 CSU graduates joining the workforce annually—half of whom come from low-income backgrounds—the fates of California's higher education institutions, economy, and society have never been more connected. However, the university faces a steep challenge. In 2017, the Public Policy Institute of California forecasted a shortfall of 1.1 million bachelor's degrees in California by 2030.[3] Closing this shortfall is imperative to maintaining the state's global position.

To address this looming degree shortfall—and continue to fulfill its service mission—the CSU launched Graduation Initiative 2025.[4] The goals of this initiative are to increase graduation rates for all students, essentially double the four-year graduation rate, and close equity gaps between Pell Grant–eligible students and underrepresented minority students and their peers. To achieve these goals, the

CSU is tackling barriers to student success both in and out of the classroom. One barrier the CSU seeks to eliminate is the prevalence of food and housing insecurity.

Hierarchy of Needs

Maslow's hierarchy of needs is a highly referenced psychological framework, often used in education to describe the motivation of an individual.[5] In short, Maslow asserted that people are motivated to obtain certain needs and that some needs take precedence over others. A person can have the capability to move *up* the chain toward a level of self-actualization (i.e., live up to their full potential); however, failure to meet lower-level needs restricts progress. Therefore, not all people will move through this hierarchy in a linear manner; many will oscillate back and forth between different types of needs.[6]

Maslow grounds this hierarchy in the idea of first meeting our most basic needs for physical survival.[7] For example, priority needs require the meeting of physiological demands, followed by meeting safety needs, obtaining love and belongingness, acquiring esteem needs, and acclaiming self-actualization. Therefore, a person acts to meet the next set of needs not yet/currently satisfied. Applying Maslow's theory to addressing basic needs in higher education aligns with the general idea that a student's lack of access to necessities will hinder progress, self-efficacy, and the ability to move up the hierarchy to achieving and maximizing their talents and potential.

Maslow's hierarchy is consistent with the experiences of students who lack the necessities. When students face uncertainty related to nightly shelter and meals, they often experience increased stress, anxiety, and wellness concerns. Furthermore, as these students often lack the ability to attend class, focus on their coursework, or study for exams, college completion rates are affected. Due to its close link with student success, the CSU has become a national leader in researching and addressing food and housing insecurity in higher education. The CSU's leadership on basic needs stems from a commitment that begins at the very top.

Institutional Change

Since arriving at the CSU in late 2012, CSU chancellor Timothy P. White has worked to ensure that every student receives the holistic support needed to be successful. During visits to all 23 campuses, Chancellor White met repeatedly with faculty, staff, and students, including those experiencing food and housing insecurity. In addition, data gathered by CSU campuses led directly to greater insight in the challenges and obstacles that too many college students—in the CSU and elsewhere—face as they progress toward their lifelong dream of earning a baccalaureate degree. The combination of first-person experiences and data became the impetus for the CSU Basic Needs Initiative.[8] The initiative soon undertook a system-wide analysis of policies, practices, programs, and services related to food and housing insecurities.

In 2015, Chancellor White commissioned a snapshot study, entitled *Serving Displaced and Food Insecure Students in the CSU*, to understand better the breadth of food and housing insecurity facing students at a single CSU campus.[9] The following year, the CSU spearheaded and funded an even more robust and comprehensive system-wide survey regarding basic needs of students at all 23 campuses. Conducted by Drs. Rashida Crutchfield and Jennifer Maguire and described in detail in the next chapter, the 2018 Study of Student Basic Needs provided a comprehensive analysis of four-year college students who experience food and housing insecurity. Outcomes demonstrated that 20 percent of CSU students experienced *low food security* (diminished nutritional quality) and an additional 21.6 percent experienced *very low food security* (reduced nutritional quality and diminished nutritional quantity—hunger).[10]

Drs. Crutchfield and Maguire announced the results at the second CSU Basic Needs Initiative Conference in February 2018.[11] The conference served as a catalyst to the CSU's current commitment to heighten awareness, education, and on-the-ground action related to food and housing insecurity. Conference attendees analyzed the results of the study, shared best practices and research opportunities, and developed statewide partnerships and programs to further address food and housing insecurity.

Balancing the responsibilities of attending college (e.g., tuition and fees, academic preparedness, completion of coursework) while sustaining their basic needs is a challenge many college students experience. It is not a new challenge. In fact, on most campuses, staff and faculty can point to colleagues who keep a cabinet full of food in their office for students, or who serve as the point of contact for community resources. Faculty and staff are familiar with the college student experience, which too often includes poor eating habits, lack of nutrition, and limited financial resources that do not stretch to the end of the month.

As awareness of the breadth and depth of the problem continues to grow, and as the impact of food and housing insecurity on student success becomes more apparent, higher education institutions must evaluate how university communities view these obstacles and how they respond. Simply put, universities must implement institutional change.

Every institution of higher learning is unique. Students are unique. While cookie-cutter models of change can inform action, they often do not allow campuses to embrace their differences and align with their respective campus cultures. True transformation occurs when university leaders recognize that change is necessary and intentionally engage the overall organization in creating a shared vision.

Within the CSU, a call by Chancellor White was key in transforming organization culture system-wide. On all campuses, research, practice, shared leadership, and collaboration have led to action plans focused on supporting all students in their path to a college degree, including addressing their basic needs. Chancellor White also called for a collective response, organized through the system office and led by the newly created position of director of the Student Wellness and Basic Needs Initiative. This response includes the development of a framework for the CSU Basic Needs Initiative, the coordination of champion change agents, and advocating for policy change through the state legislature. This multilevel response drives institutional change at the CSU.

Framework

The successful application of a basic needs framework will likely begin with two assumptions: (*a*) the university recognizes that some attending students have ongoing unmet needs, such as needs related to food and housing insecurity, and (*b*) the campus is ready to assist these students. To address basic needs in a higher education setting, a multipronged approach recognizing five key areas is recommended: (1) address the *immediate needs* of students, (2) facilitate the *growth* of campus-based basic needs services and the number of students who can access these services, (3) *scale* best practices from one campus to others, (4) *collaborate* with partners to expand impact, and (5) ensure long-term *sustainability* of basic needs services.

Through the Basic Needs Initiative, the CSU is working to address students' basic needs by implementing this framework to reach students and connect them with food and housing resources.

Immediate Needs

In the wake of the 2015 snapshot survey,[12] CSU campuses took significant action to meet the immediate needs of students. This is often considered the "triage" stage of helping students in crisis. Campuses established the foundation of basic needs programs and services, with the purpose of developing a "safety net" to address immediate crises and intervene within a shortened time frame.

For example, all CSU campuses currently utilize a food pantry or food distribution program. A nexus point has thus been created for students to connect to—and learn about—various programs, services, and resources that can help alleviate food insecurity challenges. A number of campuses have emergency housing programs available for students who find themselves in need of short-term housing. Several campuses have implemented a case manager model with a point person responsible for contacting students in crisis and connecting them with available resources, either on or off campus. Additionally, many campuses have developed websites and other collateral to provide information to students regarding food and housing resources.

Growth

In this second area, the CSU Office of the Chancellor is working with campuses to track promising practices and identify gap areas in order to grow the campus's basic needs services to reach additional students. Focus has been placed on building connections between campus departments to ensure a seamless flow of information and support to students.

In June 2017, California governor Jerry Brown signed into law Senate Bill 85. This legislation allocated $2.5 million to the CSU for campuses to receive "Hunger-Free Campus" designations.[13] The CSU leveraged these funds for greater impact by creating a request for proposals. This process allowed campuses to apply for funds to either enhance or develop additional supports to address food and housing insecurity among students. Funds were distributed based on strategies the campuses committed to implementing and the number of students being served.

Among other actions, campuses will use these funds to develop and enhance food pantries, create or expand a system where students can donate unused meals from a meal plan, and designate a campus point of contact knowledgeable about CalFresh (California's federally funded Supplemental Nutrition Assistance Program [SNAP], which provides healthy and nutritious foods to low-income individuals meeting income eligibility rules) who can help students with the application process.

Scale

The CSU Office of the Chancellor is developing strategies to scale single-campus best practices system-wide. For example, the Office of the Chancellor has partnered with CSU Chico's Center for Healthy Communities (CHC) on the first-ever higher education system-wide effort to conduct CalFresh Outreach (CFO) with students on college campuses. For the current CFO cycle, CSU Chico works with 19 CSU campuses to increase CalFresh awareness, help eligible students apply for CalFresh, and partner with local county social service offices to identify and reduce barriers associated with program enrollment. The goal is to continue looking for ways to increase access to these services and expand services to engage all 23 campuses in CalFresh activities.

Collaboration

The Basic Needs Initiative includes a focus on partnerships with other California higher education institutions. The Higher Education Alliance is a network of allies formed between the California Community Colleges (CCC), the University of California (UC), and the CSU to work collectively to spearhead efforts statewide and prioritize the implementation of and advocacy for basic needs resources for students across the state.

Collaboration on basic needs efforts also exists *within* the CSU. The California State Student Association (CSSA), the CSU Academic Senate, and the CSU Alumni Council have identified the

Basic Needs Initiative as an important strategic focus. The CSU is working closely with all groups to facilitate discussions and action regarding the basic needs of students. A system-wide Basic Needs Advisory Committee is being established, which will include students, faculty, staff, and administrators from different departments and sectors. The advisory committee will regularly meet and discuss ways to address food and housing insecurities among students.

Additionally, the Office of the Chancellor has begun to have key conversations with federal and state agencies regarding the implementation of Electronic Benefit Transfer (EBT) resources on CSU campuses. EBT programs allow students to use CalFresh benefits to purchase healthy food while on campus. The CSU, CCC, and UC are also working with the California Department of Social Services (CDSS) to more efficiently and effectively deliver services, specifically CalFresh, to college students statewide.

Sustainability

Sustainable programming is essential to the long-term success of the Basic Needs Initiative. As such, the CSU must act innovatively to expand the continuum of care, not only reaching students who ask for help but also identifying and reaching students who may be reluctant to speak up. Faculty and staff awareness of the absence of basic needs must be raised. Faculty and staff must be informed as to how to identify and direct students who may need resources.

Another aspirational strategy is to integrate basic needs screenings into on-campus health center visits, so that when students call to make an appointment, they are asked whether they are currently experiencing food or housing insecurity. Health center staff should be appropriately trained to support these students and connect them with resources. Within this area of sustainability, there will be a focus on research and evaluation, as the use of data-driven results is necessary to implement innovative strategies.

Case Studies

Since the CSU began its focus on addressing students' basic needs, campuses have seen great success. These successes have been phenomenal to watch, evolving from tiny, unfunded concepts to brilliant partnerships and collaborative efforts by campus, community, and statewide leaders.

California State University, Chico: SNAP/CalFresh
Fall 2018 Enrollment: 17,488

CSU Chico's CHC has been a successful Prime CFO Contractor since 2009 and has provided training and technical assistance to over 100 college campuses throughout California. This is the first university system–wide effort to conduct outreach for CalFresh utilizing a student peer-to-peer model on college campuses. The CHC CFO team works alongside the CDSS and local county social service departments to provide eligibility information, application assistance training, and innovative outreach practices specific to the high-need student population. These trainings support drop-in assistance and CalFresh Outreach events, eligibility prescreening, and application assistance on each campus to increase CalFresh participation and access to healthy food among students and their families.

The key to CHC's CFO success has been the collaborative development of best practices for universities and colleges. These strategies include the integration of CFO into other campus-based basic needs programs such as campus food pantries, partnerships with community food banks, campus meal plans, fresh produce vouchers, farmers' market EBT promotion and tastings, campus pop-up pantries, department-specific fieldwork internship placements, nutrition education workshops and demonstrations, outreach promotions in the classroom and during academic advising, and incorporation of food assistance language and competencies within campus curricula. For example, CHC's campus team provides drop-in assistance five days per week at the Hungry Wildcat Food Pantry location. Students can receive immediate short-term food assistance in addition to CalFresh application assistance as a means of long-term support. A high level of student engagement is ensured through promotions within various student service departments (e.g., financial aid, student health centers, admissions, and Educational Opportunity Programs).

California State University, Sacramento: Case Manager Model
Fall 2018 Enrollment: 31,131

> When students are clothed, fed, sheltered, and have a sense of belonging, they can continue to focus on their success and timeliness to degree. Students whose needs are met quickly and effectively are less likely to drop out, or extend their college plans. When the administration fully understands this and fully supports interventions to address this, the campus culture shifts and people are able to tie in these efforts to the overall mission of the university.
>
> —Danielle Muñoz, basic needs case manager

CSU Sacramento employs a unique case manager model to reach students facing food insecurity. Referrals by members of the campus community to the case manager allow this case manager to follow up with a licensed clinical social worker who utilizes a trauma-informed approach to address students who may need assistance meeting basic needs. This high-touch approach boasts a strong success rate for supporting students in crisis.[14]

In order to spread awareness of this resource, Sacramento State is dedicated to outreach and education. For example, through the use of academic department meetings, faculty learn about the food insecurity case management model and engage in a discussion about how to spot early warning signs of need and how to make appropriate referrals. The university also engages the support of students and staff from programs around campus, including resident advisors, academic advisors, peer mentors, members of student government, career counselors, disability counselors, library staff, and more. The campus communications department works to highlight case management efforts and leverage the campus-wide "Monday Briefing" to remind campus community members of available services.

The philosophy behind the integration of the case management strategy is threefold:

1. The single-point-of-contact model was chosen, as it encourages referrals by being user-friendly for the campus community. Most people do not feel equipped to make an assessment of students' basic needs; therefore, the ability to refer to a professional case manager removes the fear associated with independently assessing these needs. In addition, with today's need for faculty and staff to wear multiple hats and balance multiple time-consuming commitments, the simple task of referring a student to the case manager is both a timely and accurate way to appropriately support students. Campus community members are thus encouraged to be approachable, aware, and responsive in order to refer students to available resources. The case manager possesses the clinical skills necessary to quickly and appropriately support students.

2. The case manager must be able to conceptualize a complex case holistically, unpack the various concerns of the case, and empathize with and connect to students in order to develop a feasible plan to address each (often moving) aspect of a student's circumstance. The case manager must have a working knowledge of the full array of supports and resources available on and off campus, while being intimately familiar with the various eligibility criteria for each. Even one referral to an inappropriate resource may undermine trust, especially with students in crisis with elevated emotions.

3. Follow-up and follow-through are crucial to ensuring success with this strategy. When students are in crisis, their executive functioning is often not at its best. While a referral may seem straightforward, a student in crisis may not have the organizational skills and follow-through required to pursue that referral. The resource may seem beyond their immediate reach. This approach, therefore, depends on a case manager who believes in recurring and timely follow-up with students. This follow-up often serves as the difference between a successful referral and a continuing problem. In many ways, the case manager serves as the student's own executive functioning until the acute crisis is managed.

Sacramento State's primary method of engaging students is through a "see something, say something" mantra followed by faculty, staff, and student leaders. Rather than relying solely on self-referrals, there is a reliance on others to notice when support is needed. Each summer, Sacramento State invests many hours in trainings for peer mentors, orientation leaders, resident advisors, and student leaders. These trainings have led to a high volume of referral calls and emails that allow the university to continue to foster a culture of care. When incorporated into "see something, say something," members of the campus community feel inclined to report what they see and refer those in need. Every call or email is returned. The only way to really create a lasting shift in the campus culture is to demonstrate that every student case deserves attention.

The keys to success at Sacramento State have been the encouragement and utilization of collaboration, a campus culture of care, and a single-point-of-contact model. Teamwork across campus has led to successful efforts, such as emergency housing, SNAP outreach, intern programs, a student emergency fund, a professional clothing drive, and more. The support of the university administration was a catalyst for changing the campus culture. When campus administration recognizes that academic success is closely linked to students' fulfilment of basic needs, that realization, combined with training, outreach, and consistent response, encourages student support and assists in student success, retention, and higher graduation rates.[15]

California State University, Fresno: Fundraising
Fall 2018 Enrollment: 24,995

CSU Fresno's on-campus food pantry, known as the Fresno State Student Cupboard, received a tremendous outpouring of donor support from alumni, corporate partners, community members, faculty, staff, and students. When the Student Cupboard opened in November 2014, Fresno State's president, Dr. Joseph Castro, allocated one-time funds to kick-start the project.

Shortly after opening, however, it became evident to campus leadership that because of the size and scope of student need, the Student Cupboard would require ongoing funds to sustain itself over the long term. In March 2016, Fresno State launched a unique fundraising campaign, March Match-Up, where private donors matched funds raised by the campus community. While not affiliated with the national collegiate basketball tournament, Fresno State's March Match-Up campaign took advantage of the renewed attention and school spirit that the sporting event garners each year.

The campaign was a success. In 2016, the Student Cupboard raised more than $106,000, with $50,000 matched by private donors. The following year, Fresno State boosted its fundraising efforts, raising $184,475, including $82,000 in match donations. In 2018, more than $150,000 was raised—with $45,000 matched— to further strengthen the long-term viability of this vital on-campus food pantry.

In addition to generous donor support, the Student Cupboard relied heavily on campus outreach to foster buy-in from students, faculty, and staff. With strategic social media and web presence, tabling at campus events, and outreach at new student orientation, for example, Fresno State fostered a vibrant culture of acceptance and support from the larger campus community.

During the reveal event for the 2018 March Match-Up, a Fresno State student shared his powerful story about the support he received from the Student Cupboard while waiting for financial aid funds. While visiting the Student Cupboard, the student learned about other resources on campus, like dining hall meal vouchers. The student attributed the support he received from these resources, including the Student Cupboard, to helping him earn a bachelor's degree.

The success of Fresno State's Student Cupboard and March Match-Up campaign is a result of the hard work and dedication of the campus community and leadership. The money raised *only* supports the Student Cupboard. The dollars help to purchase food and hygiene items, pay for meal certificates, and pay for student assistant staffing (five students) for the Student Cupboard. Most of the food is purchased from the Community Food Bank, which provides a greatly discounted rate, helping to stretch funds.

Humboldt State University: EBT in Dining Services
Fall 2018 Enrollment: 7,774

Humboldt State University (HSU) is the first college/university in California and second in the country whose dining services offer EBT on campus. EBT provides eligible individuals, including many students, the ability to purchase food using federal government benefits through the US Department of Agriculture (USDA).

The EBT implementation plan at HSU began as a multitiered approach that involved outreach across the campus community and integration alongside the CalFresh and OhSnap! Student Food Programs.[16] As participation in CalFresh outreach efforts and participation grew on campus, it became apparent to faculty and staff that some students found it difficult to use this resource during long days spent on campus attending classes or studying.

The leadership of the University Center and dining services at HSU responded by bringing EBT services to campus. Staff and administrators from these areas worked with the USDA to understand eligibility qualifications, updated point-of-sale and accounting processes, and provided appropriate training to staff in the campus-based store. Through their efforts, the campus market gained the ability to accept EBT, but USDA rules prohibit the purchase of prepared or hot food items, limiting its use in dining halls or campus restaurants.[17]

Dining services has seen increased usage of EBT during lunch and dinner meal times. EBT sales at the campus market are around 5 percent of total store sales activity, confirming the existing need. "To me this is not just a dollar amount, but it shows that we are helping a lot of our students," said Dave Nakamura, executive director of the HSU University Center.[18]

Students who sign up for CalFresh are now notified of the EBT campus location. The campus has also worked with the county to open the campus market as an EBT location for the surrounding community. Using EBT gives students and others who might otherwise go the whole day without eating the ability to have a much-needed meal on campus.

San Diego State University
Fall 2018 Enrollment: 34,881

The Community College Equity Assessment Lab at San Diego State University (SDSU) conducts research, training, and assessment on homelessness and housing insecurity in community colleges through data provided by the Community College Success Measure.[19]

SDSU's research has identified a number of obstacles that affect student persistence and retention in community college. For example, students facing food insecurity were less likely to perceive a sense of belonging from faculty. As a result, the impacted students' presence in the classroom was not as significant, and they ultimately did not believe they belonged in college.

These findings—among others—by SDSU highlight the importance of having conversations on how to best support students experiencing food and housing insecurity as related to their sense of belonging. Armed with these findings, SDSU researchers are leading efforts to identify cultural humility and bring more awareness to food and housing insecurity, particularly in marginalized communities. These efforts—led by SDSU—are changing the assumptions and stereotypes students may experience when facing food and housing insecurity.

Researchers at SDSU also continue to expand on and share research findings across the country, publishing recommendations on how higher education leaders can better address food insecurity and engaging in equity-focused discussions regarding college students facing food and housing insecurity. These recommendations include reducing the costs associated with college, organizing a campus-specific strategy, developing vital and timely interventions, and reenvisioning how institutions award and distribute financial aid.[20]

Lessons Learned

Throughout the course of its research on basic needs and efforts to address food and housing insecurity, the CSU has identified several "lessons learned" that are applicable both to its 23 campuses and at colleges and universities across the country.

- Focus attention on both preventative measures and triage strategies

Higher education writ large must be more proactive in focusing attention on both preventative measures and triage strategies. As part of this proactive approach, colleges and universities must work to end the stigma surrounding food and housing insecurity, which negatively hinders the institution's ability to identify and support its most vulnerable students, who are often too embarrassed or scared to self-identify as needing assistance.[21] Instead, the goal of every university focused on tackling basic needs challenges should be to create a culture of inclusion and support for students from all backgrounds and circumstances, including those facing food or housing challenges.

- Evaluate and assess effectiveness of basic needs programs and interventions

In theory, opening a food pantry on a college campus is effective. A student enters the pantry with little or no food and leaves the pantry with a bag full of necessities for the week (sometimes longer). A similar statement may also be made regarding meal swipe donation programs on campus. A student speaks with staff providing oversight to the meal donations, completes the appropriate paperwork (as needed), and is immediately connected to meals. Both of these practices, among others, connect food resources in real time to students in crisis. However, the ability to assess and articulate the effectiveness of these "theory-turned-practice" strategies is lacking.

Evaluation of any program is crucial in order to present measurable impact and meaningful progress toward intended outcomes. Also important is the ability to show which program components are failing to meet intended goals and/or how those programs can be improved. A sense of urgency to meet students' immediate needs often left little time to organize a fully scaled and thoughtful evaluation plan.

A clear lesson learned has been the need for a comprehensive assessment as a part of the initial plan. This should be in place before beginning program development, implementation, and intervention. This is particularly critical because food insecurity among college students is now on the radar of the nation's leaders. This interest will no doubt lead to an increase in requests for data related to the effectiveness of interventions. Higher education institutions would do well to be ready for these requests with a comprehensive evaluation plan.

- Identify existing resources and allies

Administrators must be knowledgeable about resources available at the local, state, and federal levels. Community agencies, social services, and organizations that address food and housing insecurity in the surrounding community are natural allies. Students may not be aware of, or take advantage of, existing programs and services, so it is incumbent on campuses to make those connections for students.

At the same time, administrators must identify, nurture, and leverage partnerships—both on campus and off. At the CSU, students have proven to be deeply committed to the issue of basic needs and strong partners in the initiative. CSSA is a nonprofit, nonpartisan advocacy organization for CSU students. They expressed their concern and commitment to food and housing insecurity through a resolution entitled "Calling on All 23 CSU Campuses to Develop a Student-Centered Food Pantry and CalFresh Advising" in May 2016.[22]

The group has advocated for food and housing insecurity assistance, speaking to legislators and campus constituents and lobbying in Washington, DC, and Sacramento, California. Their work and focus have assisted with the critical need to orchestrate an organizational shift in the CSU through student empowerment and grassroots movement. As stated by CSU student trustee emerita and former CSSA president Maggie White, "We've worked to engage students by talking about the issue constantly, and chipping away at the stigma. We've also invited students to speak at committee hearings before the state legislature to share their experiences grappling with food and housing insecurity. That's been very effective for spreading the message and creating awareness at all levels."[23]

- Coordinate efforts with external partners

Collaborative partnerships among California's higher education stakeholders have helped shine a spotlight on the prevalence of food and housing insecurity across the state. Engagement now exists between the UC, CSU, and CCC through the California Higher Education Basic Needs Alliance. Through routine contact to discuss campus practices and efforts to advocate for policies and legislation, the alliance is advancing its shared agenda to the benefit of all California college students. Furthermore, the CSU continues to leverage participation in work groups, higher education collaboratives, research, meetings with social services organizations, and legislative hearings to address the issue of housing and food insecurity in higher education.

Conclusion: Next Steps

As the CSU works system-wide to ensure that all students have the opportunity to be successful, its commitment—both at the campus level and as a system—to addressing the basic needs of students is unwavering. The CSU is committed to placing mental health and student wellness at the forefront of their student-centric efforts. To once again quote Maggie White, "The next step in this movement is incorporating mental health. If you don't have decently nutritious food to eat or a safe place to sleep, you can't be as focused on your studies as you'd otherwise be. If you're struggling with your mental health and there aren't enough resources or the appropriate resources for you to access on campus, that's also a huge barrier to success."[24]

Moving forward, the CSU's Basic Needs Initiative will become more integrated as a well-being strategy to holistically serve students on their path to graduation. At the same time, the CSU will continue to foster, support, and grow campus-based programs to reach more students, scale best practices system-wide, collaborate with internal and external partners, and take actions to ensure long-term sustainability, while continuing to be innovative in the ways we support student success.

Notes

1. Raj Chetty et al., "Mobility Report Cards: The Role of Colleges in Intergenerational Mobility" (working paper no. 23618, National Bureau of Economic Research, July 2017), https://doi.org/10.3386/w23618; Michael Hout, "Social and Economic Returns to College Education in the United States," *Annual Review of Sociology* 38, no. 1 (2012): 379–400, https://doi.org/10.1146/annurev.soc.012809.102503; Philip Oreopoulos and Uros Petronijevic, "Making College Worth It: A Review of the Returns to Higher Education," *Future of Children* 23, no. 1 (2013): 41–65.

2. California State Department of Education, *A Master Plan for Higher Education in California: 1960–1975* (Sacramento: California State Department of Education, 1960).

3. Hans Johnson, Marisol C. Mejia, and Sarah Bohn, "Will California Run Out of College Graduates?," Public Policy Institute of California, Oct. 2015, https://www.ppic.org/publication/will-california-run-out-of-college-graduates/.

4. "Graduation Initiative 2025," California State University, https://www2.calstate.edu/csu-system/why-the-csu-matters/graduation-initiative-2025/Pages/default.aspx.

5. Abraham H. Maslow, "A Theory of Human Motivation," *Psychological Review* 50, no. 4 (1943): 370–96.

6. David M. Brookman, "Maslow's Hierarchy and Student Retention," *NACADA Journal* 9, no. 1 (Mar. 1, 1989): 69–74, https://doi.org/10.12930/0271-9517-9.1.69; Linda Darling-Hammond, *The Flat World and Education: How America's Commitment to Equity Will Determine Our Future* (New York: Teachers College Press, 2010).

7. Abraham H. Maslow, *Motivation and Personality* (New York: Harper & Row, 1954).

8. "CSU Basic Needs Initiative," California State University, https://www2.calstate.edu/impact-of-the-csu/student-success/basic-needs-initiative.

9. Rashida Crutchfield, *Serving Displaced and Food Insecure Students in the CSU* (Long Beach: California State University, Office of the Chancellor, Jan. 2016), https://presspage-production-content.s3.amazonaws.com/uploads/1487/cohomelessstudy.pdf?10000.

10. Rashida Crutchfield and Jennifer Maguire, *Study of Student Basic Needs* (Long Beach: California State University, Office of the Chancellor, Jan. 2018), https://www2.calstate.edu/impact-of-the-csu/student-success/basic-needs-initiative/Documents/BasicNeedsStudy_phaseII_withAccessibilityComments.pdf.

11. "2018 CSU Basic Needs Initiative Conference Addressing Basic Needs in the CSU: Supporting Student Success," California State University, https://www2.calstate.edu/impact-of-the-csu/student-success/basic-needs-initiative/Pages/Conference.aspx.

12. Crutchfield, *Serving Displaced and Food Insecure Students*.

13. "Hunger-Free Campus Designation," California State University, https://www2.calstate.edu/impact-of-the-csu/student-success/basic-needs -initiative/Pages/hunger-free-campus-designation.aspx.

14. Ronald E. Hallett and Rashida Crutchfield, "Homelessness and Housing Insecurity in Higher Education: A Trauma-Informed Approach to Research, Policy, and Practice," *ASHE Higher Education Report* 43, no. 6 (2017): 7–118, https://doi.org/10.1002/aehe.20122; Ronald E. Hallett, Rashida M. Crutchfield, and Jennifer J. Maguire, *Addressing Homelessness and Housing Insecurity in Higher Education: Strategies for Educational Leaders* (New York: Teachers College Press, 2019).

15. Crutchfield and Maguire, *Study of Student Basic Needs.*

16. "OhSNAP! Student Food Programs," Humboldt State University, http://hsuohsnap.org/.

17. "What Can SNAP Buy?," US Department of Agriculture, https://www .fns.usda.gov/snap/eligible-food-items. For more information on SNAP, see chap. 10.

18. David Nakamura, interview with author, May 2018.

19. See https://cceal.org/.

20. J. Luke Wood, Frank Harris III, and Nexi R. Delgado, *Struggling to Survive—Striving to Succeed: Food and Housing Insecurities in the Community College* (San Diego, CA: Community College Equity Assessment Lab, 2016), https://cceal.org/food-housing-report/.

21. Aydin Nazmi et al., "A Systematic Review of Food Insecurity among US Students in Higher Education," *Journal of Hunger and Environmental Nutrition*, June 22, 2018, 1–16, https://doi.org/10.1080/19320248.2018 .1484316.

22. California State Student Association, "Resolution Calling on All 23 CSU Campuses to Develop a Student-Centered Food Pantry and CalFresh Advising," May 6, 2018, https://www.calstatestudents.org/wp-content /uploads/2017/08/05-08-16-Resolution-Regarding-Student-Centered-Food -Pantries-and-CalFresh-Advising.pdf.

23. Maggie White, email to author, May 2018.

24. Maggie White, email to author, May 2018.

[8]

Research as a Catalyst for Positive Systemic Change

JENNIFER J. MAGUIRE AND RASHIDA M. CRUTCHFIELD

Editors' Prologue. Research—including the iterative process of systematically gathering and analyzing information, translating it for different audiences, disseminating it to key stakeholders, and engaging in a collaborative process—is a key strategy in the fight to end hunger and basic needs insecurity on college campuses. This chapter provides a model of publicly engaged scholarship from the perspectives of two professors and their student, staff, administrative, and legislative colleagues. It provides critical insights for scholars seeking to make connections among research, policy, and practice, as well as anyone who wants to engage with researchers to help enact systemic change. The prior chapter explains some of the institutional changes stemming from the approach to research described in this chapter.

About the Authors. Jennifer J. Maguire is an associate professor in the Department of Social Work at Humboldt State University, which is the northernmost campus in the California State University. She has worked collaboratively with students, scholars, practitioners, and community members on a variety of innovative research and projects to help transform how students' basic needs are met in the California State University, as well as inform state policy being redesigned to better serve students in higher education. Previously she worked for the California Department of Health and Human Services as a child welfare social worker, where she worked closely with foster youth and former foster youth navigating the transition to adulthood.

Rashida M. Crutchfield is an associate professor in the School of Social Work, California State University, Long Beach. Dr. Crutchfield led Phase 1 of the California State University Office of the Chancellor study on food and housing security and was co-principal investigator for Phases 2 and 3. She came to this work as a former staff member of Covenant House California, a shelter for youth experiencing homelessness.

This chapter aims to provide campus activists and scholars a framework for working together in robust partnerships that benefit students. Less about specific research, this chapter focuses primarily on the use of research as a strategy or intervention to enact change and serve students and the colleges and universities they attend. As an example of how research can be used as an approach for systemic change, we discuss a study we led together entitled the California State University (CSU) *Study of Student Basic Needs*,[1] which was funded by the CSU Office of the Chancellor. The study documents the prevalence of food and housing insecurity among CSU students and its effects on student success. This study served as a foundation for research-driven systemic change that helped mobilize coordinated efforts, program development, and policy advocacy. It was the groundwork for what has become the CSU Basic Needs Initiative (BNI),[2] discussed in the prior chapter by Drs. Denise Woods-Bevly and Sabrina Sanders. Beyond the BNI, others used the research to further coordinate campus and community initiatives across the system. To demonstrate how strategic partnerships between researchers and stakeholders facilitated program development and policy advocacy toward the elimination of college student hunger, we invited leaders in the movement to share their perspectives on the process. We close the chapter by synthesizing some of the lessons we learned along the way that may be useful for other future partnerships with researchers.

The Early Days: Motivation to Study Basic Needs Insecurity and How We Were Trying to Address It with Research
Rashida Crutchfield's Perspective

As a researcher, I bring my own perspectives on and incentives for conducting a study of basic needs, and I chose to specifically focus on homelessness early on because of my personal and professional experiences. Prior to academia, I was a practicing social worker, primarily focused on community organizing, intercommunity dialogue, and policy advocacy. From 2004 to 2007, I was employed at Covenant House California, a shelter for homeless and runaway youth. There I interacted with a number of residents who were attending college and confronting obstacles that had less to do with their own challenges living with homelessness and more to do with the policies and structures of college institutions that did not seem to be prepared for their needs. For instance, one resident, a bright and academically prepared young woman, was refused access to her financial aid because she did not have access to her parents' tax forms. She was told, "You don't look homeless. You're probably just fighting with your parents." Many staff at the shelter advocated for her and resolved the issue, but I wondered, "What is happening for others?" At the time, there was no research on the collegiate homeless experience, and my passion was born.

I recognize that my training as a social worker influences my work as an academic from both micro and macro vantage points. I consider it my responsibility to avoid bifurcating who I am as a social worker and an educator in how I work collectively with staff, faculty, and administrators on campus. It is often easy for faculty to stay distant from student affairs or presume to be the imparters of knowledge for staff. One of my roles with staff and administrators from across the 23 CSU campuses has been to honor the expertise of my peers at all levels, to seek to know their perceptions and expertise, and to bridge connections that may not currently exist. While I share research, I also validate, encourage, and support those who work directly with students in many different capacities whenever possible.

From a macro perspective, I am fully aware of how meaningful it is to have the opportunity to use research to effect change. When I entered academia, I worried that I had "sold out" or distanced myself from critical community work to seek equity for marginalized communities. Contributing to the research, amplifying the voices of students, influencing policy, and finding answers and options in response to the question "What is happening for others?" are absolutely the best ways I can think of to make a career.

My dissertation included a study of 20 community college students who were all experiencing homelessness, shelter, or transitional living. Presenting that research on my campus raised the awareness of the then CSU, Long Beach (CSULB), provost David Dowell and our campus president Jane Conoley. Both expressed support for my work and a strong intention to address these issues on our campus. Provost Dowell introduced me to the CSU Office of the Chancellor, which was already moving to allocate funding for this study. Conducting Phase 1 of the CSU study opened statewide conversations about the need to support our students in ways many had not yet thought about.

President Conoley supported the leadership of our then dean of students Dr. Jeff Klaus to bring together campus stakeholders to establish what is now called the CSULB BNI.[3] As an active member of this committee since its inception, I have provided expertise as a researcher and social worker. We developed an emergency grant program, a meal-sharing program, emergency housing, and collaborative links between on- and off-campus services. We have also supported the work of the student government, Associated Students Inc. (ASI), in developing our campus food pantry. The CSULB BNI has always incorporated the work of social workers, social work students, and student development fellows to ensure that students are responded to in a way that honors their experiences and addresses their needs with appropriate care. The ability to build a career that both links resources that directly support the needs of students and amplifies the voices of students through research grounds me firmly in my ideal vision of what professional academic life should be.

Jennifer Maguire's Perspective

Initially, I gravitated toward this work as a person with insider knowledge and experience in growing up poor, finding my way to college, and then struggling to pay for it. The experiences of living on the edge for so long were exhausting and nearly unbearable. However, I survived, and with my PhD I landed a tenure-track faculty position. I thought that the struggle was behind me, but, frankly, the memories stayed with me. I wish I could have pressed "skip" or "fast forward" on some of them, but the lessons were indelible and made it impossible for me to ignore the students whom I encountered who were navigating their own struggles. However, being an assistant professor came with more power, privilege, and responsibility than I anticipated. In my new role, I felt accountable to students to learn more about whether basic needs insecurity was a widespread experience and why it was so severe.

In fall 2013 I began working with colleagues on this issue, and we identified a grant partnership with the Humboldt County Department of Health and Human Services that had the potential to provide funds for paying students to conduct peer-to-peer outreach about CalFresh, California's iteration of the Supplemental Nutrition Assistance Program (SNAP) on campus. We received funding, and the award made it possible to hire eight students. These students started generating "a buzz" about CalFresh, and from there many partnerships emerged, and with it students' access to healthy food increased. This was the beginning of OhSNAP! Student Food Programs,[4] which now serve as the hub for campus-wide initiatives to support students in meeting their basic needs.

We also talked with campus stakeholders. It became clear that although many people felt empathy for students facing food and housing insecurity, there was a belief that the problem was unique to a few students and that addressing their unmet basic needs was not the responsibility of higher education. As one administrator stated, "It sounds tough, but we are not a welfare agency." These types of comments inspired early assessment to demonstrate that student hunger was not a personal problem but a systemic one, so we surveyed students at Humboldt State University (HSU). This survey later served as the pilot of the CSU *Study of Student Basic Needs*. In 2015, I received a message from Dr. Crutchfield to be a participant in Phase 1 of the CSU study. We reconnected a few months after the interview, and our collaborative work began with Phases 2 and 3. Since then, I have had the privilege to engage with talented and committed leaders in ways that have created opportunities to continue to work toward discovering and creating better supports for students.

CSU *Study of Student Basic Needs*:
A Tool for Positive Change

A higher education degree is one of the greatest opportunities for long-term economic stability, a pathway toward asset growth, and debt management.[5] Alongside this opportunity is a popular narrative of the "starving student," held and perpetuated by many—the idea that students might be mismanaging their money and, as a result, eat lots of noodles to make ends meet. Contrary to this common notion, empirical evidence suggests that too often students do not have enough financial means to cover the cost of college and living expenses for a range of reasons, least common of these being personal budget mismanagement. Not having enough money takes a heavy toll on their well-being and ability to earn a higher education degree. CSU *Study of Student Basic Needs* research was initiated for a variety of reasons, including interest by the CSU Office of the Chancellor to address basic needs insecurity among students as a part of CSU Graduation Initiative 2025 (GI2025),[6] which has the following goals: "GI2025 is the California State University's ambitious initiative to increase graduation rates for all CSU students while eliminating opportunity and achievement gaps. Through this initiative the CSU will ensure that all students have the opportunity to graduate in a timely manner according to their personal goals, positively impacting their future and producing the graduates needed to power California and the nation."

In our roles as educators, researchers, and social workers, we had our own ambitions for this research. Although our priorities were closely aligned with GI2025 goals, we were also concerned about the health and well-being of students. We had both conducted prior research on basic needs insecurity and wanted to expand the research to provide evidence to support or repute the anecdotal stories we heard from students that pointed to the potential need for systemic changes to better support students. We wanted changes to be informed by research-driven recommendations that came from both students and higher education experts.

Theoretical Frameworks for the CSU Study

The CSU *Study of Student Basic Needs* was also informed by strong theoretical bases. Theoretical frameworks help provide lenses as we conceptualize the study of marginalized communities, remaining consistently responsive to the truth of students' words and experiences.

Maslow's hierarchy of needs postulates that access to fundamental needs influences overall opportunity.[7] We start from the most basic of assumptions that all students need adequate nutrition and housing in order to be healthy and perform well. Further, cumulative advantage and disadvantage theory is used to help explain how early advantages and disadvantages shape life opportunities and have cumulative impacts over time.[8] Students entering college with a history of being underresourced during earlier life experiences may navigate significantly more hardships while working toward a degree than those students with more advantages. These frameworks support the position that providing access to emergency responses while also developing longer-term policy solutions related to basic needs and college affordability may increase the odds of future successes for students, such as completing their university degrees and flourishing in the labor market.

As researchers with employment history as social work practitioners, we place strong personal and professional emphasis on a strengths-based perspective that suggests that while it can often be easier to focus on the problems and challenges of certain populations—often people of color, low economic status, or both— it is of vital importance to assess for capabilities, knowledge, and experiences of all people.[9] Furthermore, we consider how policies, systems, and access to resources may influence outcomes. While this perspective does not encourage dismissing obstacles and disadvantages, it promotes strongly integrating assets versus deficits into research and practice.

Validation theory also provides a theoretical perspective for our work. Validation theory incorporates both the efforts of the student as a participant in her own experience and the institution's active role in engaging and supporting her. Rendón theorized that first-generation students, low-income students, and students of color have more difficulty transitioning into college.[10] Students may express doubt about their capabilities to achieve in college and are less likely to be aware of the need to take advantage of opportunities for support, such as faculty mentorship or support services. Since students who are basic needs insecure share many attributes of housed students who are impoverished, this theoretical frame is used. This theoretical frame is fundamental to the BNI and its study, as it acknowledges that our individual campuses and our system as a whole have a responsibility to retain marginalized students, researching the perspectives of students, staff, faculty, and administrators to enhance the responsiveness of institutions to addressing these needs.

Aware that homelessness and food insecurity can carry stigma, many students may purposefully hide their circumstances and be unwilling to discuss their difficulties with those who are able to help.[11] Given that students are sometimes unwilling to divulge their experiences and are hesitant to seek support,[12] we suggest that it is the responsibility of institutions to develop opportunities and systems for outwardly engaging students, versus waiting for students to take the lead in accessing support. From this perspective, students have the self-determination and the ability to make personal choices and decisions that influence their lives and determine their own success and failure. However, validation theory requires that the student is not the sole proprietor of success and redirects the focus from the individual to the interaction between the individual and outside systems.

The CSU Study

In February 2015, Timothy White, of the CSU Office of the Chancellor, commissioned Dr. Rashida Crutchfield to conduct Phase 1, entitled *Serving Displaced and Food Insecure Students in the CSU*.[13] The study shed light on how CSU campuses were meeting the needs of housing and food insecure students and offered recommendations to ensure academic success and graduation for these students. On the system-wide level, Phase 1 provided a mixed-methods study from the perspective of CSU staff, faculty, and administrators about their observations of food and housing insecurity and campus support programs that were in place to help students. Phase 2 of the study was motivated by the need to describe basic needs insecurity and effects on academics, physical health, and mental health from students' perspectives. In 2016, Phase 2 of the CSU *Study of Student Basic Needs* commenced and aimed to explore the prevalence, scope, and health impacts for CSU students who experienced very low food insecurity and homelessness and to learn more about coping methods and supports students used.[14] A survey was distributed to a census sample across all 23 CSU campuses, with 5.8 percent participation (N = 24,537). The sample was largely representative of the student body. Student participants volunteered and were selected for focus groups and interviews based on reported levels of homelessness and food insecurity from the survey. Interview and focus group data were collected at 11 CSU campuses with students (n = 213) who identified as housing insecure, food insecure, or both on the quantitative survey.

We found that 41.6 percent had experienced food insecurity in the past 30 days. Nearly 22 percent of those reported very low food security, meaning that they were not getting enough food, linked with hunger; were experiencing weakness, difficulty concentrating, and sickness; and were missing school. African American and first-generation students (66%) were far overrepresented when compared with the CSU student average. Tiffany from Long Beach State shared what very low food security was like for her: "So basically what I used to eat three days out of the week was like Minute Maid and chips and that'd be it. . . . I wouldn't eat anything 'cause I didn't have any money." Far different than some might have anticipated, Tiffany was not an outlier; we heard this type of story many times throughout our research. The national prevalence rate for food insecurity among US households in 2016 was 12.3 percent (low and very low food security combined), making the case for college students emerging as a new food insecure population of concern.[15]

It is important to note that food insecurity rarely occurs in isolation. Though continued research is needed to clarify correlations between food insecurity and issues of housing insecurity, poverty, educational cost, living wage, and affordable living, it is clear from this research that students experience a multiplicity of hardships while striving to earn a university degree. Further, those hardships have compounding consequences for their overall well-being.

In our survey, we also found that 10.9 percent of CSU students had reported being homeless in the past 12 months. African American and first-generation students were a disproportionally represented group, with nearly 18 percent having reported experiencing homelessness. Elizabeth from Fresno State University shared this about her experience with homelessness: "And so, I ended up being homeless for about four months. Sleeping on friends' couches, staying in my car." She had budgeted just fine for the year, but she was pushed out by higher rent rates. She did not budget for a new deposit and first and last months' rent and ended up leaving school.

Aware that our institutions strive for student success and retention to graduation, it was important to move beyond prevalence and explore how these issues are related to academic achievement. We found that the more food insecure or homeless a student, the lower their reported grade point average and higher their level of academic concerns, such as anxiety about academics, work, trouble concentrating, and time management. With regard to physical and mental health indicators, we found that the more food insecure or homeless a student, the more likely that student was to have experienced symptoms of poor mental and physical health in the past 30 days, as well as missed more days of school or work. For students who experienced very low food security, homelessness, or both, they reported often missing nearly double the days of school or work because of poor physical or mental health symptoms when compared with their secure peers.

The research findings demonstrated that the crisis was widespread and persistent. Additionally, findings from research at public two-year and four-year institutions were key in identifying that basic needs insecurity was pervasive across public higher education. This was the momentum needed to launch the BNI, a multipronged effort to systematically work toward meeting the basic needs of students through research and data-driven decision-making, system-wide coordination, community partnerships and collaboration, and policy advocacy and legislation. We knew that confining our role to conducting the research was not enough and that disseminating information and engaging stakeholders at many levels would promote data-driven program and policy development.

Multidimensional Perspectives from Stakeholders on How Research Can Be Used as an Approach to Systemic Change

The role of faculty researchers in enacting systemic change can be critical. Faculty can collaborate with stakeholders, leveraging their research skills to amplify the stakeholders' voices. We define "stakeholders" as those who are affected by basic needs insecurity or are involved in support of solutions that work toward its amelioration. In this case, they are staff, faculty, students, administrators, community agencies, policy advocates, and legislators engaged in forward movement in this work. Findings from the CSU *Study of Student Basic Needs* informed system-wide program and policy recommendations that aid the fight to end hunger and homelessness among college students. Without a community of talented individuals from diverse backgrounds who are working at a variety of touchpoints in the system, the research would not lead to change. Though there are instances when our work is presented to amplify the perspectives of those we work with and to address food insecurity, we also asked them to provide their own narratives to inform and engage others in this movement for change. Thus, we invited those with whom we have worked closely to tell how they used findings and recommendations from this study as a platform to keep basic needs initiatives focused on ending hunger and homelessness among college students. Each person described how the study has been a powerful tool for engaging and developing allies, advancing promising programs and services, and developing policy change.

Voices of Students: The Role of Research in Promoting Grassroots Change

Maggie White, Master of Public Administration
California State University, Stanislaus
2017–18 President of the California State Student Association (CSSA)
Currently, CSSA Legislative Policy Analyst

Students had been talking about being hungry and homeless for a long time, and some campuses were beginning to be active in addressing these concerns, but there had never been an organized approach to tackling these issues system-wide. While students were expressive of their needs and unafraid to advocate for attention to be paid to these issues, we could largely provide only anecdotal evidence as to what we were experiencing on our campuses as students who went to class and worked hard but were unable to make ends meet as we attempted to progress toward our degrees. The CSU *Study of Student Basic Needs* provided a legitimacy to stakeholders outside of the CSU and a platform for students, particularly those experiencing basic needs insecurity, to raise their voices and advocate for tangible solutions. The study and its researchers set the foundation for a true partnership between stakeholders by including students from the very beginning in disseminating findings to a variety of audiences. This partnership empowered students to tell their stories, backed up by significant findings from the research study, and really made an impact in their conversations with legislators, administrators, and members of the public. Suddenly, everyone was talking about the importance of basic needs, through a student-centered focus that was respectful, nonexploitative, and solution oriented.

CSSA had prioritized basic needs security as a top issue for which to advocate throughout the 2017–18 year, based solely on student leaders' perspective of the issue as one that was serious and deserving of immediate attention. While campuses had begun to open food pantries and establish short-term resources for students experiencing homelessness, there had not been a concentrated systematic conversation about these issues and how best to tackle them. The research provided by the CSU *Study of Student Basic Needs* created a larger platform than we could have created alone because it involved all stakeholders and brought fresh data from each campus to the attention of decision-makers. This enabled students to back up their personal stories with hard numbers, which I believe swayed legislators to consider the issue with a greater sense of urgency. Suddenly, what students had been saying about being homeless and hungry was backed up with data, and it became very real for the people who had not experienced it for themselves.

In the long term, I believe that this research has set the foundation for continued partnership between faculty, students, and administrators when it comes to other issues that affect student success. This research created the space at the state level for students' voices to be amplified, and these stakeholders being on the same page in regard to basic needs insecurity created a wave of activism that swept the state and resulted in never-before-seen levels of awareness around the issue, as well as support from legislators that likely would not have occurred without students' voices and faculty's research progressing hand in hand.

Chant'e Catt, Bachelor of Sociology Graduate
    and Master of Social Work Student
Humboldt State University
President and Founder of the HSU Homeless
    Student Advocate Alliance

In countless meetings, we as members of the Homeless Student Advocate Alliance (HSAA) were told that without empirical evidence, anecdotal stories of students' struggles were just not enough for campus programs and administrators, funders, nonprofit organizations, or public agents to participate in planning to support positive change. Without reliable and relevant data, advocacy has no evidence to support its argument. Not only did the quantitative statistics highlighted in the basic needs study validate our own experiences, but the qualitative findings also humanized the numbers that proved that students were homeless and hungry.

Working with the institution, alongside professors like Dr. Maguire and Dr. Crutchfield, positively and directly affected the legitimacy of our group's efforts and helped messaging that aligned with our priorities to reach stakeholders quickly, compared with what normally would have taken students like us years. The data collected verified to key decision-makers that student homelessness and housing issues in our community were real and helped our club's "asks" to be considered. The study findings led HSAA to recommend a housing liaison for students experiencing housing insecurity. Highlighted in Phase 2 of the BNI study is point 4: "Incorporate staff as single points of contact who are trained in trauma-informed perspective in programmatic responses to students experiencing food and housing insecurity and co-locate space for the contact and student."[16] Because both our student group and the institution's study had similar findings, our club's advocacy was heard, and soon after, the position of off-campus housing liaison was created at HSU.

Further, we have had great success in the creation of a 24-hour safe study space and an education program, the Humboldt Tenant and Landlord Coalition, created by social work students for student tenants and landlords. Additionally, we worked to discontinue on-campus housing deposits and advocate at city council meetings for new off-campus student housing developments that will offer low-barrier housing in Humboldt. Using the data from the CSU *Study of Student Basic Needs*, our club has successfully advocated for these initiatives. The study has been a bit of a handbook to us, as a point of reference to help make sure the campus is held accountable for making the necessary changes needed by students of our time.

Hawk McFadzen, Master of Sociology Student
California State University, Dominguez Hills

Food access is not just an issue that impacts me personally; it is my area of study, and a subject about which I am passionate. My advocacy is rooted in personal experience, drives every one of my scholastic endeavors, and is fueled by the input from my fellow students who are food insecure. Much of the food access literature that I draw from points to the simple act of growing fruits and vegetables as a quick and easy solution to food insecurity.[17] Therefore, throughout the 2017 calendar year, I advocated heavily for the establishment of an urban farm on the campus of CSU, Dominguez Hills (CSUDH). I feel that my proposal was met with confusion about how and why an urban farm could be vital to campus, so I remained the sole advocate for the project until fall 2017. For urban agriculture advocates, this is not a surprising interaction.[18] We are very passionate about urban farming, but it is simply not on many people's radar, especially not many people in leadership roles. The challenge became educating first about food security and how it affects our students and second about the role an urban farm could play in alleviating that problem.

The farm proposal, although gaining the support and advocacy of two key faculty and staff members (Dr. Jenney Hall in environmental studies and Ellie Perry, the sustainability coordinator), and despite having been awarded a $10,000 grant from the CSU Office of the Chancellor, remained an unapproved project. Lacking official on-campus approval meant that the project stalled and threatened to wither on the vine. The turning point appeared to be the 2018 California State University Basic Needs Initiative Conference in Sacramento,[19] where the results of the CSU study were officially released. Within a week of that conference, not only was the Campus Urban Farm approved, but the school also established a Basic Needs Task Force, of which I am a member. It is my belief that the thorough and impactful results of the research conducted by Drs. Crutchfield and Maguire provided the necessary combination of education and data to justify the establishment of an urban farm at CSUDH. It is my hope that soon we can replicate the study to specifically focus on our campus to measure the effects of the urban farm.

Carolyn Tinoco, Master of Public Administration Student
California State University, Dominguez Hills
Vice President of Finance for the CSSA

As a CSUDH student, I was invited to speak about my experiences on a panel at the CSU Basic Needs Conference, and I shared my personal story with food insecurity. At the conference, I attended workshops on solutions individual campuses had already put in place. The conference and presented research were beneficial to my campus because they showed how important it is for students to have access to healthy fresh food, a place to live, and mental health care to be successful in college. The first action CSUDH took was to provide a monthly fresh food pop-up open to all students. We now have a Basic Needs Committee that brainstorms solutions to these issues, reviewing campus successes and areas to improve.

Not only was the research important to my campus, but it also boosted my self-esteem to help me become a better leader and advocate. At the conference, the workshops I attended helped strengthen my own lobbying efforts, and I used this information to urge legislators to help fund the CSU. Now, in my current student leadership role as vice president of finance for the CSSA, I hope to keep addressing these issues until students no longer face them.

Rachael Simon, Master of Social Work
California State University, Long Beach
Homelessness Policy Fellow for the Office of Los Angeles
    County Supervisor Sheila Kuehl

During my master of social work (MSW) program at CSULB, I was given an incredible opportunity to work as a graduate research assistant on the CSU *Study of Student Basic Needs*. This role allowed me to collect and analyze qualitative data from students across

California experiencing food and housing insecurity. I am incredibly passionate about working to solve homelessness and entered the MSW program in hopes of developing the clinical skill set to best support individuals and communities experiencing poverty, housing instability, and homelessness. However, my experience as a researcher completely shifted my professional trajectory from a direct service provider to that of a community-based, policy-oriented social worker. While I love working in direct service and understand the magnitude of such work, this research experience allowed me the opportunity to bear witness to the direct correlation between research and the creation of policies that address structural inequalities and directly influence system changes. As a student, I witnessed the day-to-day changes that occurred as a result of this research and saw the tangible, significant impact it had on the lives of students struggling to meet their basic needs.

As a result of my engagement in the CSU research, I completed my MSW degree and obtained a fellowship in local government working to create policies that address homelessness in Los Angeles. Seeing the immense social justice implications of this research has been an inspiration for me to obtain a PhD in social welfare so that I may continue working to create impactful changes on systemic levels.

Stephanie Marie Valverde Loscko, Master of Social Work
California State University, Long Beach

While working toward my MSW degree at CSULB, I had the great privilege of working as a research assistant on the CSU study with Dr. Crutchfield. One of the most poignant components of my involvement in this work was conducting interviews and focus groups with participants facing food and housing insecurity. The willingness of the individuals to participate in the study in and of itself was so powerful, but to hear about their experiences firsthand was incredibly humbling. I have never been involved in work that has made me feel such an immense amount of gratitude and passion quite like this has. The social justice implications of this research feel as though they could have infinite possibilities to impact campus communities by strengthening programs and policies around food and housing security that will inevitably increase the success rate of students across the nation. Something I found so compelling about this work was the fact that qualitative research findings would be something of great importance when it came to shaping recommendations. It's amazing how often we hear about the numbers but how seldom we hear the actual story behind the statistics. The value that was set on that aspect of this work is something that contributed significantly to my aspirations to be part of it. My involvement in this study has strengthened my cognizance of how research can impact policy and serve as an important intervention as both a social worker and a citizen. It has influenced my desire to achieve a profession that involves policy advocacy and achieve my PhD. My gratitude for this experience is immeasurable, as it has greatly influenced my aspiration not only to seek a career as a social justice advocate but also to pursue a lifestyle that contributes to the betterment of communities everywhere.

Anthony Mota, Communication Major and Counseling
    and Social Change Minor Undergraduate Student
San Diego State University

I am a Guardian Scholar, a student who has been in foster care, and I have dealt with food insecurity during my time as a student at San Diego State University (SDSU). I was very fortunate to have the opportunity to tell my narrative at the CSU Basic Needs Conference and present on the work we are doing at SDSU. These opportunities have opened new doors and passions for my future. Since participating in the conference, I have been invited to participate as a student advocate for the SDSU Crisis Response Team, which includes administrators from various departments across the campus. The goal is to utilize school resources from all the different departments on campus to provide services for all SDSU students who might have issues with food insecurity, homelessness, or transportation; who are in abusive or toxic environments; or who need psychological and emotional assistance. The BNI research served to reinforce the need for these initiatives. In addition, this year I have taken on more leadership and volunteer roles on campus with the Guardian Scholars Program, including assisting my peers with filling out CalFresh, MediCal, and financial aid forms. I have also presented at workshops for foster kids in high school, with the purpose of empowering them and showing them how going to college is an option. By advocating for change and supporting my peers, I feel more empowered and connected to my campus. I am grateful for all the work the CSU has done to address issues with basic needs for all its students.

Voices of Staff: The Role of University Research in Campus Program Development

Sesley Lewis, Coordinator of Food and Housing Security
California State University, Los Angeles

As a recent college graduate of CSU, Los Angeles (CSULA), I can easily recall my experiences with food insecurity and housing instability as a student. It is also easy for me to remember the intense struggle of having to balance academics and work, while worrying about how rent was going to get paid and meals were going to be provided, not to mention the other expenses, oftentimes unexpected, that "adulting" brings. I remember looking for events on campus that would have food and being excited when someone would unexpectedly pay for lunch. I can also recall having to find the most efficient way to pay for textbooks and still have money to continuously have a roof over my head. Fellow peers would describe me as extremely involved and always busy, but they would not associate food and housing insecurity as a label of identity that reflected my daily struggle. In fact, the phrase I would hear often was "you really have it all together," which indeed was the illusion that I gave off but was not my reality. I did not speak of my struggles because I didn't want to seem as if I really didn't have it together. Why? Because I was going to figure it out. What I know now that I did not know then is that so many students are experiencing the same struggle, and some with great intensity.

The movement in support of student food and housing security has substantially grown over the past few years. I believe that this work has been tremendously impacted by the research completed through the CSU, especially the CSU BNI. The results of this work have championed campuses to eliminate food and housing insecurity by implementing programs and giving voice to students like myself. For CSULA, the research lit a fire that led to the immediate implementation of a campus food pantry, the CalFresh Outreach Center, a meal-sharing program, emergency housing, and an emergency grant program, and as a student, I was a part of the staff that helped these programs blossom. Within a year of these programs being implemented, over 3,000 students were able to receive assistance, and the work continues to grow. Prior to the CSU releasing this research, little to nothing could be found that focused on the basic needs that students so often go without. In addition, the research has brought awareness to the experiences and struggles of food and housing insecure students, and it has also provided a framework that supports and destigmatizes students experiencing these situations.

The CSU BNI research has demonstrated the need for programs and services that contribute to students' overall academic success. While I have personally lived these experiences, the study expands and sheds light on the system-wide need for programs that focus on student basic needs. This further fuels the movement toward addressing and ultimately eliminating student food and housing insecurity.

Ravin Craig, MA
Humboldt State University Health Educator

The data provided by the research done by Drs. Crutchfield and Maguire are essential to ensuring that basic needs initiatives on campus are effective, strategic, and sustainable. At HSU Dr. Maguire led the creation of OhSNAP! Student Food Programs, and without the thoughtful revolutionary research that she has done, we would not be where we are today.

Research data can provide an essential benchmark for proving that what we are doing is effective. More than that, data are necessary to identify the ways in which practices need to improve. Much of what was created and done to address basic needs issues at HSU was done without foundational data, and done as quickly as possible, because the need, anecdotally, felt so incredibly urgent. The research has shown where our initial efforts are falling short and what we need to do to move beyond reactionary action to active systemic prevention of basic needs shortfalls. Some concrete ways in which OhSNAP! has used the data collected about basic needs have been to apply for additional grant and campus funding, identify campus and community stakeholders who need to be present when creating action plans, center the voices and experiences of those who are most in need, and convince campus administrators of the urgency of many of these issues. The goal of basic needs initiatives should not be to bandage the wound, but to get to the root of the issue. Data are key to understanding the systemic nature of basic needs inequities.

The identification of gaps and the benchmarking that these data have given groups like OhSNAP! are important to creating sustainable praxis. Research data are key to creating actionable theory. The doing of work cannot happen without the knowing. The typical view of college students is changing. The CSU is at the ground level for that change. Anyone who does not view this research as an urgent call to action in higher education is not paying attention. With these data, those of us doing the on-the-ground work of basic needs support finally have a set of tools for addressing hesitance from administrators and tackling outdated institutional barriers.

Voice of an Administrator: The Role of University Research in Campus Administration

Lisa Rossbacher, Campus President
Humboldt State University

The CSU BNI has contributed to our work at HSU in three important ways. First, the research by Professors Maguire and Crutchfield has helped quantify the magnitude and extent of food and housing insecurity among our students. This information helps us all understand the issues more clearly and provides data that are helpful in articulating the situation to stakeholders—including the surrounding community.

Second, this research has motivated the university to develop short-term strategies to address students' basic needs. These actions range from hiring a housing liaison to assist students looking for safe, affordable housing to developing a smartphone app to notify the campus food pantry when food is available after an event. Since October 2016, more than seven tons of leftover food have been distributed on campus.

Third, HSU's deep commitment to social justice leads us toward systemic solutions to helping students achieve housing and food security. As a university, we are looking for long-term answers to the issues facing our students, as highlighted in this research. HSU is developing partnerships with external organizations and agencies to provide affordable housing for students. We have met with state legislators to advocate for students. We consistently evaluate our internal policies to ensure that they are as supportive as possible of students who are struggling to meet their basic needs. And the Board of Trustees of the CSU also appreciates the importance of taking a systemic approach to these issues. After learning about this research, several trustees requested that the topic of addressing students' basic needs become a regular part of every board agenda.

At the core of this research, the link between addressing basic needs and student success is fundamental. Adequate healthy food and safe shelter are vital to students' ability to focus on their studies, to learn in an appropriate environment, and to obtain the maximum benefits from their education.

Voice of a California Legislator: The Role of University Research in Legislation

Shirley Weber, PhD, MA
California Assembly Member, District 79
Chair, Select Committee on Campus Climate
Member, Higher Education Committee

For 40 years, as a university professor, I heard the humorous stories of how my students coped with the economic challenges of being a student. And while these stories were important, I felt that my only avenue was to give money from my pocket or seek scholarship funds for the student. Little did I know how widespread the problem was, or that our social service agency policies prevented simple solutions.

In 2012, when I ran for the assembly, I had a student working in my office who was doing research on a real-life problem she faced, the use of the Electronic Benefit Transfer (EBT) program, which is CalFresh, or commonly called "food stamps" on campus. I was intrigued by her stories of inconvenience and decided to remedy this program once I was elected.

During my first year (2013), the student did an internship in my office in Sacramento and helped us write my first bill to address the problem, AB 832. This bill was to simply allow EBT cards to be used on campus like credit cards to purchase meals. Boy, was I surprised by how much bureaucracy was involved in maintaining the status quo. Needless to say, AB 832 died because others felt that it was too expensive to install the machines on campuses to make use of them in our eating establishment on campus. At some point the cost to do this was listed as $250,000 per campus (later we learned that one of the campuses started the program with less than $500).

Fortunately, a report was released discussing hunger and homelessness on college campuses, and the results were shocking. This research opened the eyes and hearts of legislators and bureaucrats. How could we expect our students to succeed, or finish college in a reasonable time frame, if over a quarter of them were chronically hungry and homeless? Immediately students began to respond to the problem with campus pantries initiated by them. I had been appointed chair of the Assembly Campus Climate Select Committee to address the growing problem of racial, gender, and religious intolerance in our state schools. This committee became an ideal vehicle for addressing issues of hunger and homelessness on campus.

The hearings and research on this subject allowed me to author three successful pieces of legislation addressing the problem: AB 1747 (2016), AB 214 (2017), and AB 1874 (2018). Each bill addressed the issues of adopting EBT on campus, cooperation with local food banks to remove restrictions from campus collaborations, statewide CalFresh on campuses regardless of the local county's welfare limitations, and student housing. The bills have enjoyed bipartisan and agency support. Barriers to cooperation between agencies have been legislatively removed, and on all California higher education campuses (University of California, CSU, California Community Colleges) students are empowered to help each other with the full support of the state. Innovative programs are being implemented every year that are initiated by students, and my role has been to make sure that the state does not get in the way of progress and provides the necessary resources to end hunger and homelessness on our campuses.

Without compelling research, efforts to address this important issue would not have been as successful in such a short period of time. The legislation has given students the right and voice to demand better support from their administrators, and they are.

Recently, I attended a conference of student leaders discussing what is happening on their campuses. I am amazed and pleased with how they have challenged themselves to truly be a community of caring adults solving real-life problems. What a blessing.

Building and Leveraging Researcher-Stakeholder Partnerships

Both of us feel strongly about the need to build relationships that include diverse stakeholders to increase the system's capacity for community change. However, in higher education, we often work in discipline- and department-specific silos that make it challenging to find the time to collaborate and coordinate on a shared vision. Because the study was system-wide, it required us to work across areas to acquire approval and to collect data from varied points in the system. Working among varied disciplines with such a broad base of stakeholders was often extremely labor-intensive, but it was advantageous because relationships were formed that informed authentic research design and future practical use of the findings. Through the implementation of this study, we found people, often working on their own or in small groups, attempting to make change for students one at a time. We were able to work with them closely and support their efforts with the study findings in ways that further substantiated the need for their work to be funded and supported by their home institutions, as well as bringing their voices into the larger conversation about how to better support students.

Later, as we disseminated findings, we took time to meet with and participate in committees and work groups with representation within and across systems, including student services and government, academic affairs, housing, food services, financial aid, counseling, community resource groups, policy advocates, and many others. This was key for identifying champions for change who boldly worked with us to consistently publicize findings in ways that magnified momentum for the movement. Partnership was crucial to the launch of this movement and continues to be essential as knowledge of the work grows. In the previous section, you heard from leaders who are contributing to system-wide changes and how the role of research has played a part in their efforts. We conclude with what we have learned as researchers about collaborating with stakeholders to build momentum and speed for change.

Partnering with Students

Students are and have been the center of this work from the beginning. First, it started with the brave students willing to share their incredible stories of struggle and success in ways that brought the issue into the light. Students have been integral to the research process and program development as student assistants, as interns, and in their own research. Many of the students hired to do this work were also navigating daily life on campus, often without enough money to pay for food, housing, books, or school supplies. They provided clarity and insight into the data analysis and helped develop programs designed based on how students experienced them. Later, students organized as clubs or advocacy groups, and through student government, and used the findings to substantiate the need for action in ways that increased student access to healthy food and safe affordable housing. Based on what we have heard many times from students, being involved in this work had the unexpected effect of inspiring them to develop a newfound purpose and shape future career goals.

Partnering with Staff

Findings from the research generated many conversations between us as researchers and other campus program staff about promising practices that were emerging as a response to student need. More coordinated connections were made through the CSU BNI webinars and conferences aimed at sharing best practices. Frequently we heard that the research resonated with the experiences of students on their campuses and supported recommendations for creating service provision. Additionally, time and again staff shared how they were able to use findings from the study about students' experiences to leverage funding to create and sustain new programming for basic needs.

Partnering with Administrators

In many cases, there was initial skepticism from some university administrators. Although there were many instances where the stories of individual students were emotionally moving, some administrators found it hard to believe that this was a widespread issue. This idea ran against notions of the starving student narrative of the past, normalizing life on a shoestring budget.

It was important to establish that this was a system-wide issue. For some, it felt too big of a responsibility to acknowledge the enormity of the issues without a plan to solve it. It took the courage of students speaking out and starting to share their stories, trailblazing staff and administrators, and the enthusiastic support of CSU chancellor Timothy White. Once there was emphasis and resources targeted to gather data, it became easier to acknowledge the issue at the campus level. Chancellor White's show of support for research efforts demonstrated that there would be system-wide support for campuses identifying the extent of students' basic needs insecurity. The research provided a foundation to ground movement forward and guidance for next steps that campus advocates could use to feel confident about before jumping into action.

Partnering with Legislators

Separately and together, we have worked with California legislators as national advocates to advance policies that support addressing the lack of basic needs for students. In some cases, that has included data analysis that grounds the development of bills, or meeting with legislators and legislative staff to prepare them. We have provided testimony in committee in efforts to pass bills that support increased access for students, including California Assembly Bill (AB) 1930, which provides clarity regarding students' CalFresh eligibility. We also supported AB 801 to give priority registration for students experiencing homelessness and designate homeless and foster youth student liaisons to assist with financial aid and access program and fee waivers for enrollment stipulations. Additionally, California Senate Bill 85 has given state funding to support "hunger-free campuses," and these are all movements in a positive direction.[20] We continue to view this work as a crucial part of our roles as educators and researchers.

Partnering with the Public

Neither of us intended to be media mavens in this work, and that responsibility had never appeared in our job descriptions. However, reframing the starving student narrative to encourage more progressive thinking about the needs of students required that we engage with media at many different levels. After Phase 1 of the study, Rashida was contacted by reporters from both local outlets and national outlets such as National Public Radio and *Rolling Stone* magazine, and the media frenzy continued after Phase 2, with frequent meetings with reporters. Learning by doing, we had to create a concise, compelling message that would prompt audiences to get involved at social, political, and financial levels. Since then, both of us have had an active role in spreading the message, grounded in research, to expand the community of change.

Conclusion

Conducting research provides the basis for development of change on many levels, but beyond developing and implementing research, academics can be the linchpin in providing campus activists a framework for working together to benefit students. The CSU *Study of Student Basic Needs*,[21] funded by the CSU Office of the Chancellor, documented the prevalence and consequence of food and housing insecurity among CSU students and served as a foundation for research-driven systemic change that helped mobilize coordinated efforts, program development, and policy advocacy. As researchers, we have committed to supporting the leveraging of academic research for practical and political supports for students, toward the elimination of college student hunger.

Notes

1. Rashida Crutchfield and Jennifer Maguire, *Study of Student Basic Needs* (Long Beach: California State University, Office of the Chancellor, Jan. 2018), https://www2.calstate.edu/impact-of-the-csu/student-success/basic-needs-initiative/Documents/BasicNeedsStudy_phaseII_withAccessibilityComments.pdf.

2. California State University Office of the Chancellor, "CSU Basic Needs Initiative," accessed July 5, 2018, https://www2.calstate.edu/impact-of-the-csu/student-success/basic-needs-initiative.

3. "Student Emergency Intervention and Wellness Program," California State University, Long Beach, http://web.csulb.edu/divisions/students/studentdean/emergency_grant/.

4. "OhSNAP! Student Food Programs," Humboldt State University, hsuohsnap.org.

5. Jennifer Ma, Matea Pender, and Meredith Welch, *Education Pays 2016: The Benefits of Higher Education for Individuals and Society* (New York: College Board, 2016), https://trends.collegeboard.org/sites/default/files/education-pays-2016-full-report.pdf.

6. "Graduation Initiative 2025," California State University, https://www2.calstate.edu/csu-system/why-the-csu-matters/graduation-initiative-2025/Pages/default.aspx.

7. Abraham H. Maslow, "A Theory of Human Motivation," *Psychological Review* 50, no. 4 (1943): 370–96.

8. Dale Dannefer, "Cumulative Advantage/Disadvantage and the Life Course: Cross-Fertilizing Age and Social Science Theory," *Journal of Gerontology* 58, no. 6 (2003): 327–37.

9. Karen Kirst-Ashman and Grafton Hull Jr., *Understanding Generalist Practice* (Belmont, CA: Thomson Brooks / Cole, 2006).

10. Laura Rendón, "Validating Culturally Diverse Students: Toward a New Model of Learning and Student Development," *Innovative Higher Education* 19, no. 1 (1994): 33–51; Laura Rendón Linares and Susana Muñoz,

"Revisiting Validation Theory: Theoretical Foundations, Applications, and Extensions," *Enrollment Management Journal* 5, no. 2 (2011): 12–33; Patrick Terenzini et al., "The Transition to College: Diverse Students, Diverse Stories," *Research in Higher Education* 35, no. 1 (1994): 57–73.

11. Jarrett Gupton, "Campus of Opportunity: A Qualitative Analysis of Homeless Students in Community College," *Community College Review* 45, no. 3 (July 2017): 190–214; William Tierney and Ronald Hallett, "Social Capital and Homeless Youth: Influence of Residential Instability on College Access," *Metropolitan Universities* 22, no. 3 (Jan. 2012): 46–62.

12. Laura Rendón, "Community College Puente: A Validating Model of Education," *Educational Policy* 16, no. 4 (Sept. 2002): 642–67.

13. Rashida Crutchfield, *Serving Displaced and Food Insecure Students in the CSU* (Long Beach: California State University, Office of the Chancellor, Jan. 2016), https://presspage-production-content.s3.amazonaws.com /uploads/1487/cohomelessstudy.pdf?10000.

14. Crutchfield and Maguire, *Study of Student Basic Needs*.

15. Alisha Coleman-Jensen et al., *Household Food Security in the United States in 2016* (Washington, DC: US Department of Agriculture Economic Research Service, 2017), https://www.ers.usda.gov/webdocs/publications /84973/err-237.pdf?v=42979.

16. Crutchfield and Maguire, *Study of Student Basic Needs*.

17. Meleiza Figueroa, "Food Sovereignty in Everyday Life: Toward a People-Centered Approach to Food Systems," *Globalizations* 12, no. 4 (Aug. 2015): 498–512, https://doi.org/10.1080/14747731.2015.1005966; Benjamin P. Goldstein et al., "Contributions of Local Farming to Urban Sustainability in the Northeast United States," *Environmental Science and Technology* 51, no. 13 (July 5, 2017): 7340–49, https://doi.org/10.1021/acs.est .7b01011; Julia Laidlaw and Liam Magee, "Towards Urban Food Sovereignty: The Trials and Tribulations of Community-Based Aquaponics Enterprises in Milwaukee and Melbourne," *Local Environment* 21, no. 5 (May 2016): 573–90, https://doi.org/10.1080/13549839.2014.986716.

18. Debra J. Davidson, "Is Urban Agriculture a Game Changer or Window Dressing? A Critical Analysis of Its Potential to Disrupt Conventional Agri-food Systems," *International Journal of Sociology of Agriculture and Food* 23, no. 2 (2017): 63–76; Laidlaw and Magee, "Towards Urban Food Sovereignty"; Kristen E. Okamoto, "'It's Like Moving the Titanic': Community Organizing to Address Food (In)Security," *Health Communication* 32, no. 8 (Aug. 2017): 1047–50, https://doi.org/10.1080/10410236.2016.1196517.

19. "2018 CSU Basic Needs Initiative Conference Addressing Basic Needs in the CSU: Supporting Student Success," California State University, https://www2.calstate.edu/impact-of-the-csu/student-success/basic-needs -initiative/Pages/Conference.aspx.

20. For more information on policy efforts, see chap. 10.

21. Crutchfield and Maguire, *Study of Student Basic Needs*.

[9]

Amarillo College

Loving Your Student from Enrollment to Graduation

RUSSELL LOWERY-HART, CARA CROWLEY, AND JORDAN HERRERA

Editors' Prologue. Addressing food insecurity on campus should not occur in a vacuum. It is important to consider the whole student and their needs. With this perspective, the goal is to ensure that students are able to cover all of their basic material needs so that they can concentrate on learning. This chapter highlights one institution, Amarillo College (AC), that has developed an integrated, wraparound approach to student basic needs security, including food security. Over time, not only has AC launched an office on campus focused on students' material needs, fully staffed by social workers, but it has also taken an approach that addresses students' academic needs. As this book is being written, AC is engaged in a randomized encouragement trial to measure the effects of their program and services on student retention and graduation rates.

About the Authors. Dr. Russell Lowery-Hart, president of Amarillo College, was selected into the inaugural class of the Aspen Presidential Fellowship for Community College Excellence, a rigorous, executive leadership program focused on higher education reform led by the Aspen Institute and Stanford University. His leadership on poverty and culture change was featured in the June 2018 issue of the *Atlantic*.[1] Russell and his Amarillo College colleagues are focused on improving student success through systemic approaches to food insecurity and other poverty barriers. He was named the National Academic Leader of the Year for 2014. He received his PhD from Ohio University, MA from Texas Tech, and BS from West Texas A&M University.

Cara Crowley currently serves as vice president for strategic initiatives at Amarillo College. Her leadership focuses on leading institution-wide initiatives targeting a systemic approach to poverty, as well as creating a data ecosystem that drives policy and process reform addressing poverty barriers hindering student success. Ms. Crowley received her MBA, MS in history, and BS in business management from West Texas A&M University.

Jordan Herrera serves as the director of social services at Amarillo College. She coordinates and manages the services in Amarillo College's Advocacy and Resource Center, which include social services, a scholarship program, a food pantry, and the campus clothing closet. Each one of the services directly serves at-risk students experiencing barriers to their education. In addition, she supervises university social work interns and serves on many community boards and committees that directly impact Amarillo College students. Jordan is a licensed master social worker. She holds an associate degree in psychology from Amarillo College and a bachelors and masters in social work from West Texas A&M University.

Veronica found herself pregnant, and the father of her child was headed to prison.[2] She started hunting for jobs. She could never get an interview for the jobs that interested her. They required a degree. She did not have one. As a first-generation, Hispanic student, Veronica was scared to come on the Amarillo College campus. However, she knew she needed to provide a new life for her yet-to-be-born daughter. She parked her car at Amarillo College twice but did not even get out of the car. On the third trip, Veronica found the courage to get out of her car and make her way to the desk taking applications. The process was full of words she did not understand. She looked around, trying to find solace in the fact that many of the students in line looked like her—several with babies and kids in tow. At this vulnerable moment, Veronica needed a friend, some hope, and some help. Through systemic reforms to services, processes, professional development, and even the college culture itself, Veronica found the help she needed to start her educational journey at Amarillo College.

Students attending Amarillo College, as well as other community colleges across the country, define the future of our country and its ability to overcome the debilitating effects of poverty in our communities and nation. Today's community college student is dramatically different from the "traditional" college student of the past. She is often the first in her family to attend college, has children or supports other family members, works multiple jobs for minimum wage, and requires financial aid not only for tuition and books but also to cover basic living expenses. As Veronica stood in line at Amarillo College, she was seeking solace from a familiar face.

As the Amarillo College president, I am ultimately responsible for ensuring that excuses do not derail my college's ability to be more creative, effective, and efficient as we serve our students and community. Realizing that many of today's college students either attend or did attend a community college is critical to understanding the challenges these students face in higher education. Today's college student looks like Veronica. Today's student *is* Veronica. And Veronica is remarkable. She demands our attention. She deserves our support. Veronica holds the future of my community's economic success. Community college students, like Veronica, hold America's economic growth in their hands.

Understanding the Needs of Our Students

In 2011, the City of Amarillo came together to address our growing poverty rates and decreasing educational attainment. Together these educational, business, and community leaders established a community alliance called No Limits No Excuses, establishing a citywide goal of making pathways to postsecondary credentials and living wage employment accessible for all individuals.[3] At the same time as the city was conducting its data assessment, Amarillo College launched a data discussion to understand campus-wide our student course success rates and overall completion numbers.[4] What we learned shocked us. Our students were not completing their academic courses successfully. They were not graduating or transferring to a university. Amarillo College was failing our students and our community. We were a contributing factor to the lack of educational attainment in our area and its bleak economic outlook.

In addition to the data discussion, Amarillo College interviewed and surveyed our students to determine what was keeping them from being academically successful. As a former faculty member, I expected that the student responses would focus on academic underpreparedness, the need for more tutoring services, and the need for more intensive advising support systems. What I was not prepared to learn was that poverty and its challenges were the reasons our students at Amarillo College were struggling with academic success.

The results of the student surveys and interviews indicated that the top 10 reasons students identified for academic struggles had nothing to do with the classroom.[5] Food insecurity was the single greatest barrier our students identified as impacting their classroom and academic achievement. They also identified utility payments, housing, childcare, transportation, legal services, and health care as barriers hindering their academic success. Each of these 10 barriers is entrenched in poverty and its challenges. None of the barriers were a traditional "academic" barrier. The top 10 barriers to student success identified by our students changed Amarillo College, transformed our leadership philosophy, and revolutionized my focus as a college president.

As part of our college reformation, Amarillo College adopted a No Excuses philosophy based on Damen Lopez's No Excuses University Model, developed in 2012.[6] We became the first higher education partner for this network of schools committed to student success. At the heart of Amarillo College's No Excuses philosophy is a belief that we, Amarillo College faculty/administrators/staff, will evaluate all reasons for students' success and failure and remove institutional barriers hindering students' academic achievements. Amarillo College refuses to use any excuse that opens the door for a student to fail. Through our commitment to the No Excuses model and its philosophy, Amarillo College experienced a culture shift, driving us to embrace a culture of caring for students and each other—a culture of caring that loves our students from enrollment to graduation.

Creating a Culture of Caring

At Amarillo College, we identify our typical student each fall term based on student demographics. We refer to her as Maria. And I want you to meet her. She is a first-generation college student, meaning that neither parent earned a bachelor's degree or higher. Why is this significant? Maria often does not understand college terminology, processes, or the financial aid system. Over 70 percent of Amarillo College students are first-generation students. Maria is female, representing 65 percent of enrolled students. She is Hispanic. In fact, 46 percent of all Amarillo College students are Hispanic. Amarillo College is a minority-majority institution, with 54 percent of our students classified as minority. Per the Wisconsin HOPE Lab survey of our students, 54 percent of all Amarillo College students are food insecure.[7] Maria works, on average, two part-time jobs and has at least one child. Maria, at the average age of 27, is like the overwhelming majority of our students living in the war zone of poverty. As such, Maria drives our decision-making at Amarillo College. We are designing a college experience for her. We are designing a college system that understands who our students are and what their needs are today as they navigate life barriers and academic struggles. We are designing a college system that embraces a culture of caring for Maria and all Amarillo College students.

Amarillo College employees must embrace a culture change for higher education where students drive decision-making. The foundation of our culture change is rooted in our college values. Students crafted them, and college leadership and our Board of Regents polished and finalized them. These values are devoid of traditional academic "buzzwords." However, these values truly represent the purpose of our college and the commitments and behaviors our students desperately need from us. The Amarillo College values clearly identify students as the core purpose of our work.

Amarillo College Values

Amarillo College creates a No Excuses philosophy through actions, which display the following values:

1. Caring through WOW
   - Every student and colleague will say "WOW, you were so helpful, supportive, and open" after an interaction with us.
   - Every student will experience WOW through engaged, learner-centered classroom experiences.
2. Caring through FUN
   - We will find ways to have fun with each other and celebrate each other.
   - We will find ways to make our work fun and effective.
   - We will find ways to provide enriching learning experiences.
3. Caring through INNOVATION
   - We will see ourselves as a "roadblock remover" for students and for each other.
   - We will always look for ways to help others and improve our processes.
   - We will develop and implement original and creative teaching strategies.
4. Caring through FAMILY
   - We will find ways to show we care about our students and each other.
   - We will readily and effectively share information with each other.
   - We will approach our interactions with each other with trust and openness.
   - We will put the needs of others before our own.

- We will enhance learning by creating an atmosphere of mutual respect.
5. Caring through YES
   - We will think "yes" first and find solutions rather than stating "no."
   - We will be passionate about our jobs and helping each other.
   - We will promote critical thinking and problem-solving skills in curricula.

These values are written into every job description for all employees. The first item in every single job description is "serve students." Meeting and knowing Maria is the foundation of new employee and faculty orientation. Poverty competencies are woven into most faculty and staff developments. Our faculty, staff, and administration are evaluated on their job effectiveness and the manner in which they exhibit these values in executing their duties. Merit pay is connected to fulfilling these values. The work has been difficult and certainly controversial. However, our students deserve no less from the college and the employees who define it.

As a result, Amarillo College has created a true culture of caring. Whether our employees station themselves at key places in the college during registration to assist students through our processes, greet students in the parking lot and walk them to their first class, or care for our students' children during a finals week study session, Amarillo College employees care and are changing the culture of our college and community.

Creating a "Culture of Caring" requires careful systems. For Amarillo College, fall and spring general assemblies are critical. The college closes, and employees come together to gain a better understanding of our students, review our report card data, share new ideas, meet with local employers, and recognize "superheroes" who have gone above and beyond the call of duty. These meetings allow the college to provide a "Student Success Certification" for all employees.

Rebecca was able to experience the culture of caring. When her car battery needed a jump, she was comfortable asking for assistance from the first college employee she found. She often had college employees walking her to class and encouraging her stellar academic achievements.

Jamie sent a note of appreciation to the Advocacy and Resource Center after she completed her developmental education courses in the summer of 2017, expressing her love for Amarillo College and the care she received on campus. "I appreciate you helping me through the spring and summer. Thank you for the food and test vouchers. I wouldn't have started the fall without your help."

Creating a Bold Vision

In 2015, Amarillo College launched its No Excuses 2020 strategic plan and made equity and poverty one of five overall college priorities.[8] We were starting to build infrastructure for addressing poverty and food insecurity barriers. However, we knew that students held the key to our own reformation. We asked a group of student "secret shoppers" and follow-up focus groups to tell us how a college should be designed to ensure their success. Students identified relationships and customer service as the single most important issue in helping our first-generation and low-income students graduate and/or transfer.

I gathered a diverse group of college leaders, faculty, and staff to look at local and national companies, as well as educational institutions, known for strong customer service. Together, we highlighted their projects and programs that provided exceptional service to their customers. I then asked our students to help us define what exceptional customer service looks like at Amarillo College as we love our students from enrollment to graduation. By examining our student data and gaining a better understanding of the life experiences of our students, we began to reimagine higher education at Amarillo College. And for us, it all started with addressing poverty barriers and systemically creating relationships.

Poverty and food insecurity used to be one of the excuses we used for student failure. We now realize that poverty is a barrier to academic success and cannot be used as an excuse for failure. As a college, we cannot be absolved of our course and college success rates simply because our students live in the war zone of poverty. Because food insecurity was the single biggest barrier to student success, our No Excuses philosophy drove us to address it. At Amarillo College, if students fail, it is because the college did not have the right person, process, or policy in place to connect and support our students. As such, we knew we had to build a systemic approach to poverty and food insecurity.

Through the work of Dr. Donna Beegle, founder and CEO of Communication Across Barriers, Amarillo College began to build a response to poverty and food insecurity.[9] We closed the college for an entire day and required all faculty and staff to complete Dr. Beegle's poverty leadership certification. Moreover, nearly 100 Amarillo College employees have earned an additional certification as a poverty coach. The results of these trainings have allowed the college to share a common understanding about the language of poverty and food insecurity.

The most significant thing we learned from Dr. Beegle's program was her categorization of four different types of poverty: situational, generational, working, and immigrant.[10] We learned that many of our processes and policies were written from a situational poverty mind-set: "If we were struggling financially, how would we react?" Yet most of our students understood life and decision-making from a generational poverty mind-set: "Life happens to me, and I do not have control of my future." We were expecting our students to proactively approach us with their needs. With a generational poverty mind-set, our students were waiting for us to reach out, connect, and lead them through our college bureaucracy.

In 2016, Amarillo College established the Billie B. Flesher Advocacy and Resource Center (ARC), which aids students as they navigate on-campus and community resources, including food insecurity, transportation, childcare, housing, and utility assistance.[11] The ARC intentionally guides students who have life barriers preventing their success in and out of the classroom. In addition, Amarillo College and the ARC work with over 60 local nonprofits, with federal, state, or private funds, to help our students meet basic life needs without which they could be hindered from reaching their educational goals. Amarillo College partners with local nonprofits that provide funds for transportation, housing, utilities, and childcare to our students. Without these external partnerships, the college would be unable to eradicate poverty barriers our students are experiencing while attending our institution.

By striving to understand Maria and her challenges, the college can be better prepared for students like Veronica. In a 2018 report, Maria's challenges were once again reaffirmed by the Basic Needs Survey results through the Wisconsin HOPE Lab. In fall 2017, 11 percent of Amarillo College students had experienced some form of homelessness within the previous 12 months, 59 percent were housing insecure, and 54 percent had low or very low food security.[12] About 72 percent of students at Amarillo College had experienced at least one of these forms of basic needs insecurity within the previous year. Nearly 8 percent had experienced all three forms of basic needs insecurity. Maria and other students throughout our college were heroic. While facing #RealCollege struggles with basic needs, they were still studying and attending classes. However, the entire Amarillo College family knew that for Maria to graduate the college would have to continue addressing the barriers she faced and address them on a larger scale.

With a bold vision of 70 percent completion by 2020, Amarillo College's No Excuses 2020 focuses on equity, expanding our cohesive system to address student poverty barriers, and reforming institutional systems to support students through relationships and strong customer services.[13] Students like Victor, who relied on Amarillo College and the ARC to help him navigate our higher education systems, stay in college and eventually graduate.

As a 33-year-old dad with two kids and a wife, Victor came to Amarillo College seeking a certificate in diesel mechanics, a highly desired credential in our community. To go to school and support his family, Victor had to work a full-time job. He found one that allowed him to work from 7:00 p.m. to 3:00 a.m. He would sleep a few hours and then go to school in our accelerated program from 9:00 a.m. to 5:00 p.m. With kids in school and a wife with serious medical complications, Victor struggled to make ends meet. He was considering dropping out of college. His family had to skip a few meals, and it made his wife's medical issues even worse. One of his faculty members used the "social service barriers" button within the Amarillo College Early Alert System embedded within faculty gradebooks. This automatically "alerted" the ARC's social workers. They called Victor to ask how they could assist him. Victor was able to use the food pantry and even access emergency funds to fix the transmission for his truck. "You guys helped us keep everything together," he said. With a simple alert and intervention, Victor stayed in college and completed his certificate. He found a high-paying job, and his wife could then refocus on her health and her own higher education journey.

Addressing Food Insecurity at Amarillo College

After completing Dr. Beegle's poverty training, faculty were relieved to learn about some of the foundational reasons for academic failure. For many, the college had misunderstood student failure and made destructive assumptions about it. The reality was that students were hungry and their hunger was misunderstood as laziness, lack of motivation, and poor academic preparation and focus.

The day after the training, college leadership met to review the training evaluation—and to pat ourselves on the back for our "courage" to require such training. The day after the training, our faculty did not meet to discuss and evaluate the training; they met to find a way to act on it. While administrators reflected, faculty gathered to start Amarillo College's first food pantry. What started as a simple email soliciting donations to start a food pantry in a supply closet has grown into six pantries across all campuses, dozens of community partners, and a systemic approach to poverty and food insecurity.[14]

While our food pantries were initially stocked and run, voluntarily, by faculty and staff, the college knew that it needed a full systemic approach. Through faculty and staff donations, community partners, grants, and a college commitment, Amarillo College opened the ARC, which is the epicenter of Amarillo College's poverty and food insecurity system. With social workers and case managers, along with the full forces of our communities' social service agency network, students have support systems in place to address their most basic needs. As a result, students can taste academic success without the pangs of hunger to derail them.

Thank you all very much. You all have been very kind. You all are angels sent by God. You are showing me who I can be from now on.

—Anthony, Amarillo College student

Support for each food pantry distribution is 100 percent donation based, and no institutional funds purchase food or household items. The Amarillo College Foundation created a donor fund where individuals and businesses can make cash donations for our food pantries.[15] Amarillo College employees also can make payroll deductions that go directly into this account to support the food pantries on an ongoing basis. ARC personnel can access the foundation account in order to support any need not met by donations from faculty, staff, and the community.

In 2013, Amarillo College launched a partnership with our local food bank, High Plains Food Bank, to buy discounted food from their vendors.[16] But to meet increasing demand, Amarillo College also formed a partnership with Snack Pak 4 Kids in 2016.[17] This organization provides backpacks with nutritious food every Friday to children in our local school district. Snack Pak 4 Kids also has food pantries in several high schools that provide food to students throughout the week. With this partnership, ARC staff can purchase food from Snack Pak 4 Kids via their wholesale vendor relationships. This allows Amarillo College to use foundation funds in greater capacity and purchase more food for lower prices.

Students can visit the food pantry twice per month and fill a reusable shopping bag that we give them. For students who need additional food assistance, ARC staff help students complete SNAP (Supplemental Nutrition Assistance Program) forms, connect them with community resources that can provide additional food resources, and offer them additional food items from the Amarillo College pantry. Students may select any item in the pantry, but ARC staff assist students with selecting items that can be combined to provide hearty meals on a budget. We also have food items that can be reheated on campus if students are in need of a quick breakfast or lunch item.

One of the items most sought by our students surprised us— feminine hygiene products. These items are expensive, and no community, state, or federal agency helps clients access them. Once we knew of this need, the ARC staff sent a college-wide email asking for donations of hygiene products. Students, who were missing classes because of their lack of these items, were relieved to find this support. In fact, several faculty and community members committed to monthly donations of these items once they knew of the reoccurring need.

After getting enrolled in her first set of classes, Veronica found a student employment job on campus. Her classes were challenging. There were words she had not heard before and assignments that challenged her own confidence. She was not sure she could be a successful student. Even while working on campus and receiving a Pell Grant, Veronica struggled to feed her family. Because her college had a food pantry, Veronica knew she was in the right place. She pushed through her insecurities. She was able to feed her daughter and herself. She persisted, and her college was there to support her every step of the way. Amarillo College embraced her in a culture of caring. Amarillo College loved her from enrollment to graduation.

Food insecurity can be devastating for students. By building a culture of caring based on a true understanding of poverty, higher education institutions can feed their students—literally and figuratively—with no excuses.

Impacts and Lessons Learned

Amarillo College's commitment to addressing the life barriers that impede academic success has certainly helped our students. Our theory of change is simple: removing life barriers and building employee commitment to service and relationships will ultimately increase student course success and completion rates. We are seeing powerful evidence that our theory of change is working. Amarillo College retention rates have improved from 49 to 65 percent. Our students are more successful in gateway classes, with success rates increasing from 65 to 75 percent. Most excitingly, student completion rates have improved over the past three years from 23 to 48 percent. We have learned that when students are hungry, they cannot learn, and when they have food security, their academic performance reflects it. For students to see such dramatic gains in a short period of time, every college employee must play an important role.

Since the inception of our poverty initiative, Amarillo College has continued to grow our project annually. In the first year, Amarillo College assisted less than 1 percent of our enrolled students with social services and food insecurity needs. Today, we have grown our project to serve well over 27 percent of our enrolled students.

During the 2018–19 academic year, the ARC aided nearly 6,000 student visits with social services. When comparing to the previous academic year, Amarillo College increased student usage of the ARC by 30 percent. Specifically, the ARC assisted over 1,000 students with addressing food insecurity needs (12% of total enrollment).

Amarillo College attributes this significant growth in students served to using data analytics to identify at-risk students, connect them to social services, and address food insecurity needs before the semester begins or as early into the semester as possible. Amarillo College uses data analytics to identify students who have multiple dependents and earn less than $19,000 annually. By identifying these students prior to the start of the term, staff in our ARC contact and work with the students to determine whether they need any financial assistance to address poverty barriers that potentially could hinder their academic performance and success in the upcoming term. By using predictive modeling to put our theory of change into action, Amarillo College has increased course success, degree attainment, and transfer success for all students.

Our data show that if students access college and community resources, they will be successful. Amarillo College and the ARC work daily to ensure that no student fears enrolling in college or fears failure. We work to ensure student success by connecting students with available resources across our campus and throughout our community. Amarillo College is committed to student success—no excuses. Amarillo College daily seeks ways to overcome the stigma surrounding poverty. We strive to assist students living in poverty with creating a new outlook on life—an outlook that removes fear and replaces it with hope, belief in oneself, and a focus on the future.

Conclusion: No Excuses 2025

Given the impact of our work on behalf of Maria already, Amarillo College cannot turn back. Because our future is tied to Maria's success, we must be more intentional, systemic, and predictive in building our system to scale. With its next strategic plan, No Excuses 2025, Amarillo College plans to achieve the following five goals related to our No Excuses Poverty Initiative:

1. We must expand the reach of our predictive analytics outreach to identify students who might be at risk and connect them to resources before they even start their first class.
2. We will build a comprehensive case management system leveraging advisors, social workers, faculty, and staff to love students from recruitment to completion.
3. We will work more effectively with our community partners to tackle food insecurity for students and their families well before they become Amarillo College students by working with our local school districts and food insecurity infrastructure. We cannot wait until they enroll to solve this crisis. We know that the earlier we address the food insecurity crisis, the more likely students will matriculate into higher education and graduate.
4. We will build a robust fundraising plan specifically for poverty issues within our student body. We must leverage community resources to tackle insecurities in food and housing, transportation, childcare, and health care.
5. Finally, we will build a robust student health center that not only meets students' food insecurity needs but also integrates these services with mental and physical health needs in an intentional and comprehensive manner.

As Amarillo College continues to refine its calling to address the poverty barriers of its students, it will continue to meet its true calling, which is loving its students from enrollment to graduation. Veronica has seen that love, knows that love, and now shares that love with other Amarillo College students who are struggling to meet the challenges of life and school one day at a time.

Veronica had challenging life barriers upon entering Amarillo College. Thankfully for her, Amarillo College was prepared for her success. "I knew I had to give my kids a different life. The ARC and access to resources like a food pantry gave me hope that other people saw potential in me and were willing to give me that little push to stay focused," she said. Had she come a few years earlier, Veronica would have been a statistic rather than finishing as the commencement speaker for the Amarillo College graduating class of 2017. She graduated from the local university a year later with a bachelor's degree in communication. She still visits the campus. She is mentoring new Amarillo College students while starting her first professional job. Veronica observed,

> *Even at my university, my AC support system stayed with me. I got texts. I still received help with food on the occasions I couldn't make everything come together. So many college employees came to my university graduation. At first, I thought they were just there for me and I started crying. Then I looked around and understood they came for so many of us. They loved us. You [the college president] say all the time, that AC employees must love students to success. You all truly loved me to success, not just at the college and through my university, but into the workplace.*

Notes

1. Marcella Bombadieri, "Colleges Are No Match for American Poverty," *Atlantic,* May 30, 2018, https://www.theatlantic.com/education/archive/2018/05/college-poor-students/560972/.

2. All student names have been changed.

3. "No Limits No Excuses: Amarillo Partners for Postsecondary Success," Amarillo Area Foundation, https://www.amarilloareafoundation.org/no-limits-no-excuses; "NLNE The Partners: Amarillo College," Amarillo Area Foundation, https://www.amarilloareafoundation.org/2017/06/30/nlne-the-partners-amarillo-college/.

4. "Poverty Initiative," Amarillo College, https://www.actx.edu/arc/poverty-initiative.

5. "Top Ten Student Needs," Amarillo College, https://www.actx.edu/arc/top-ten-student-needs.

6. Damen Lopez, *No Excuses University: How Six Exceptional Systems Are Revolutionizing Our Schools* (Argyle, TX: TurnAround Schools, 2013), 1–303; see also "What We Believe," No Excuses University, https://noexcusesu.com/about/what-we-believe/.

7. Sara Goldrick-Rab and Clare Cady, *Supporting Community College Completion with a Culture of Caring: A Case Study of Amarillo College* (Madison: Wisconsin HOPE Lab, 2018), https://hope4college.com/wp-content/uploads/2018/09/wisconsin-hope-lab-case-study-amarillo-college.pdf.

8. "Amarillo College Strategic Plan," Amarillo College, https://www.actx.edu/strategic/.

9. See https://www.combarriers.com/.

10. Donna Beegle, "Overcoming the Silence of Generational Poverty," *Talking Points* 15, no. 1 (2003): 11–20.

11. "Advocacy and Resource Center," Amarillo College, https://www.actx.edu/arc/index.php.

12. Goldrick-Rab and Cady, *Supporting Community College Completion*.

13. "Amarillo College Strategic Plan."

14. "AC Pantry Is for AC People by AC People," Amarillo College, https://www.actx.edu/arc/ac-pantry-is-for-ac-people-by-ac-people.

15. "Donate to Our Most Pressing Needs," Amarillo College Foundation, https://www.actx.edu/foundation/donate-to-our-most-pressing-needs.

16. See https://www.hpfb.org/.

17. See https://www.sp4k.org/.

[10]

Addressing Student Hunger through Policy Change

Leveraging Federal Food Benefits to Support College Completion

AMY ELLEN DUKE-BENFIELD AND SAMUEL CHU

Editors' Prologue. Public policy serves as a critical component to addressing food insecurity among college students. Poverty is a systemic issue, and food insecurity is a symptom of this unhealthy system. While it is important to address the symptoms, one cannot truly end student hunger without working to improve the root of the problem. This chapter describes the role of policy in ensuring that students' basic needs are met, including describing public benefits that can provide students with resources beyond financial aid. The authors also share a case study from the state of California illustrating the ways advocacy work can improve students' access to these types of resources. Finally, the authors offer recommendations for change in both state and federal policy.

About the Authors. Amy Ellen Duke-Benfield is a Senior Fellow at the National Skills Coalition. She analyzes and advocates for policies that better serve low-income adults and other nontraditional students in postsecondary education and training and provides technical assistance to federal, state, and local advocates and governments in these areas. Previously, she was a senior policy analyst at the Center for Law and Social Policy, where she led efforts to better align state and federal public benefits and postsecondary policies to build more comprehensive financial supports for low-income students. She directed the Benefits Access for College Completion initiative, which sought to increase access to public benefits and financial aid for low-income students at colleges across the country. She holds a BA from Swarthmore College and a master of divinity from Emory University.

Samuel Chu is the national organizer for MAZON: A Jewish Response to Hunger, leading local and regional advocacy campaigns on issues of food insecurity. He is also a fellow at the Center for Religion and Civic Culture at the University of Southern California. Previously, Samuel was the founding board chair and president of One LA-Industrial Areas Foundation, one of the largest broad-based organizing networks in the nation, and served as the first executive director of California Faith for Equality and the California Faith for Equality Action Fund. Samuel is a first-generation immigrant from Hong Kong and holds a BA in political science from the University of California, San Diego, and a master of divinity in ethics from Fuller Theological Seminary.

Americans see college as a key to economic mobility and stability. Better-educated workers earn higher wages and are more likely to be employed.[1] Those with associate and bachelor's degrees earn 31 percent and 77 percent more, respectively, than those with only a high school diploma.[2] People without postsecondary credentials will have greater difficulty getting good jobs in the future.[3] Since 2008, the year the Great Recession began, 99 percent of all jobs created in the US economy have gone to those with at least some college education, and 71 percent have gone to college graduates.[4] Higher education levels also correlate with favorable social returns such as better health and higher rates of civic participation.[5] While the economic gains to securing a postsecondary credential vary based on race and gender, they are still a good investment for individuals, families, and communities of every background.[6] Even more, without a college degree, half of the children who grow up poor will remain poor as adults. A college degree lowers those figures to one in six.[7] These are some of the most likely reasons why many more people in the United States are attending college.

However, as more students seek the financial and social returns of higher education, it is increasingly harder to attain. For students who started at four-year public institutions, the six-year completion rate for the fall 2010 cohort was 62 percent. Only two in five students who began at a public two-year college earned a certificate or an associate or bachelor's degree within six years.[8]

One of the principal barriers to more students pursuing and completing college is the lack of sufficient family income and financial aid. Over the past three decades, college tuition and fees have increased nearly four times faster than the median income and four and a half times faster than inflation.[9] During the same period, the average in-state cost for an undergraduate at a four-year public institution has nearly doubled—even after accounting for all financial aid—from roughly $8,000 in 1990–91 to nearly $15,000 in 2017–18. The net price for full-time students attending public two-year colleges also increased over that time period.[10] Thirty-one percent of college students have incomes below the federal poverty level, 53 percent have incomes below 200 percent of poverty, and 32 percent receive a Pell Grant.[11]

The rapid increase in college prices, combined with student aid funding at the federal and state levels that has not kept up, has resulted in sizable and growing unmet need. Unmet need is the gap between college costs and what a student can afford to pay through savings, grants, scholarships, and other aid that does not need to be repaid. Based on US Department of Education data from the academic year 2015–16, nearly three in four students experience unmet need. Average unmet need among all students attending two-year, public institutions is $4,920, while those attending four-year public institutions face a gap of roughly $9,100, with students of color disproportionately facing unmet need and at higher amounts than white students.[12] Students try to make up the shortfall by working more hours, attending part-time, and taking out sizable loans—all of which make completion more challenging. When these strategies do not work, they skip meals and forgo stable or safe housing.

Given these realities, it is not surprising that some college students are facing inordinate levels of food insecurity. A recent US Government Accountability Office (GAO) report on college student food insecurity found that 39 percent of all undergraduates—almost 7.3 million—are at risk of food insecurity because of low household income. The US Department of Agriculture (USDA) defines food insecurity as a lack of consistent access to enough food for a healthy life. Those individuals with low food security report reduced quality, variety, or desirability of diet, and those with very low food security exhibit multiple indications of disrupted eating patterns and reduced food intake, including skipping meals, because the household lacks enough money and other resources for food. Estimates of food insecurity among college students included in the studies the GAO reviewed ranged from 9 percent to well over 50 percent, with 22 of 31 studies estimating food insecurity rates of over 30 percent.[13]

The Wisconsin HOPE Lab's third national survey in 2017, encompassing 43,000 students at 66 institutions in 20 states and Washington, DC, found that 36 percent of university students and 42 percent of community college students were food insecure in the 30 days preceding the survey. A larger survey of community colleges in 2016 showed that 56 percent of students were food insecure.[14] The 2016 survey also found that basic needs insecurities, which include both food and housing insecurity, affect marginalized students, such as students of color and foster youth, at a higher rate and are associated with long work hours and a higher risk of unemployment. According to the authors, being food or housing secure does not impact the level of academic effort among students.[15] However, working more than 15 hours per week negatively impacts students' grades.[16] Two recent surveys of college systems in California found that 40 percent of respondents from University of California campuses and 42 percent of respondents from California State University campuses experienced food insecurity.[17]

There is a growing public understanding that student aid alone is not enough to help students fund their postsecondary aspirations.

Some students are unable to meet their basic needs with existing traditional higher education financial assistance, such as Pell Grants and state student aid. Public benefits such as the Supplemental Nutrition Assistance Program (SNAP; also known as food stamps) and the Special Supplemental Nutrition Program for Women, Infants, and Children (WIC) can help low-income students make ends meet while they are in school. SNAP is a means-tested program that provides a monthly benefit that can only be used to purchase groceries. WIC provides vouchers for nutritious foods to low-income women, infants, and children at nutritional risk. These programs can reduce unmet need by supplementing the patchwork resources students currently use, increase the financial stability of students, and help them care for their families. According to the evaluation of the Benefits Access for College Completion project, which funded benefits access demonstrations in seven community colleges, benefits access can have a positive impact on students' academic progress toward degree completion, especially for students who bundle multiple benefits while enrolled.[18]

Like financial aid programs, public benefit programs feature their own complex rules, some of which serve as a disincentive to low-income individuals attending college. Others influence whether a student can attend part- or full-time. These decisions can determine how fast a student completes college and attains family-supporting employment. Special rules limit the availability of SNAP benefits for college students unless they are working, are caring for children, or qualify for another exemption. This chapter will discuss the federal SNAP policy rules, examine the options states have to increase access for low-income eligible students, and provide examples of state policy best practices. The chapter will also briefly address federal WIC policy rules. In addition, we lay out a range of policy recommendations for the federal and state governments to address college student food insecurity.

Nutrition Assistance Programs:
Introduction and Overview
Supplemental Nutrition Assistance Program

SNAP, formerly known as the Food Stamp Program, was first created by the Food Stamp Act of 1964 and then renamed in 2008. SNAP is a means-tested program that provides a monthly benefit that can be used at stores or farmers' markets to purchase food, with the exception of alcohol, pet food, and prepared foods. To be eligible, a household's gross monthly income cannot be over 130 percent of the federal poverty level (FPL). States do have flexibility to adjust and increase the income limits up to 200 percent of FPL using broad-based categorical eligibility (BBCE). BBCE is a policy that makes most households categorically eligible for SNAP because they receive cash or a noncash Temporary Assistance for Needy Families (TANF) benefit.[19] If a household passes the gross income test, they must also pass the net income test, with a net income that is at or below the FPL, after taking into account deductions. For a family of three, the FPL used to calculate SNAP benefits in 2018 was $1,732 a month, with 130 percent of the FPL for a family of three being $2,252 a month, or roughly $27,000 a year. The income test is higher for larger families and lower for smaller families.

Unlike some other public benefit programs, such as Medicaid or the TANF program, eligibility is determined at the household level, reflecting the fact that people who live together usually prepare meals together. The SNAP benefit is not intended to pay for the entire food budget of a household, but to supplement it. At the end of 2018, the maximum monthly benefit amount for a single individual was $192 per month, and a family of three was eligible for up to $505 per month.[20] Most recipients receive less because they have some earnings or other income, or they have few expenses. The benefit calculation takes into account earnings and sometimes particular assets (many states no longer count assets at all), as well as expenses such as a portion of a household's shelter expenses and their child-care costs. According to the USDA, in fiscal year 2019, the average SNAP recipient and household received $125 and $247, respectively, in monthly SNAP benefits.[21] According to the national food bank network, Feeding America, most households run out of food and SNAP benefits before the end of the month, at which point they often seek help averting hunger at one of the 60,000 food pantries or soup kitchens throughout the country.[22]

The SNAP program is jointly administered by the USDA's Food and Nutrition Service and state governments. Except for in some states that have added their own state dollars to the program to increase benefits or cover people who are not federally eligible, SNAP benefits are fully federally funded. This means that the federal government sets the benefit levels and eligibility rules, although applications and eligibility determinations are conducted by the states and, in some cases, counties. While the SNAP benefits are federally funded, the administrative costs are shared evenly between the state and the federal government. Ten states administer SNAP at the county level: California, Colorado, Minnesota, North Carolina, North Dakota, New Jersey, New York, Ohio, Wisconsin, and Virginia. In some of these states, but not all, the county also helps to share some of the administrative costs. Households can apply for SNAP through multiple avenues, such as at public benefits offices or by mail, and most states now offer online applications and eligibility interviews over the phone, which makes it easier for those juggling work, family, and school and also for those who lack access to affordable childcare or dependable transportation to apply.[23] SNAP recipients must reapply for benefits every 6–12 months.

SNAP benefits are distributed monthly via an Electronic Benefit Transfer (EBT) card, which can be used to buy food at authorized retailers—grocery stores, but also other places that sell food, including discount stores, bodegas, and farmers' markets. SNAP generally cannot be used to buy prepared foods. If a state has a Restaurant Meals Program (RMP), then students who are homeless, disabled, or elderly may be able to purchase prepared food at approved locations.[24] SNAP cannot be used to pay for college cafeteria meal plans, but if the college cafeteria has been approved to accept an RMP, SNAP benefits may be used by a student who is homeless, elderly, or disabled to purchase a meal at that location. Students who live in residence halls and receive more than half their meals from a meal plan are not eligible for SNAP benefits.

Special Supplemental Nutrition Program for Women, Infants, and Children

WIC provides federal grants to states for supplemental foods, health care referrals, and nutrition education for low-income pregnant, breastfeeding, and nonbreastfeeding postpartum women. These grants also are used for infants and children up to age 5 who are found to be at nutritional risk. Many low-income student parents of young children may be eligible for WIC. To be eligible for WIC, applicants must meet categorical (e.g., pregnant, breastfeeding), residential, income, and nutrition risk eligibility requirements. Applicants' gross income must fall at or below 185 percent of the FPL.[25] Most states use the maximum guidelines, but states may set lower standards. Certain applicants, including those eligible to receive SNAP, Medicaid, or TANF, or in families in which certain family members are eligible to receive Medicaid or TANF, can be automatically determined income eligible for WIC even if their incomes are above 185 percent of FPL. Unlike SNAP, applicants must be seen by a health professional such as a physician, nurse, or nutritionist who determines whether the individual is at nutrition risk. In many cases, this is done in the WIC clinic at no cost to the applicant. Qualifying medical-based conditions include anemia or underweight, and a qualifying dietary-based condition includes a poor diet. WIC provided an average value of $61.24 in food per participant per month in fiscal year 2016.[26]

Depending on the state, WIC participants receive checks or vouchers or use an EBT card to purchase specific foods and beverages each month that are designed to supplement their diets with specific nutrients that benefit WIC's target population.[27] This includes foods like eggs, milk, whole grain bread, fruits, vegetables, fish, and yogurt. Benefits may also be used for the purchase of infant formula.[28] Depending on whether the individual is pregnant, postpartum, breastfeeding, an infant, or a child, an eligible individual usually receives WIC benefits for six months to a year at a time, after which the recipient must reapply.

Like SNAP, WIC is administered by the USDA Food and Nutrition Service. Unlike SNAP, which is an entitlement that must always have sufficient funds to cover those who are eligible, even when demand is up, WIC funding is considered discretionary and appropriated yearly, with no guarantee that the program will expand as a result of increased demand. Since 1997, Congress has provided sufficient funding to cover all eligible applicants.[29]

Research has shown that WIC supplemental foods provide wide-ranging benefits, including longer, safer pregnancies, with fewer premature births and infant deaths; improved dietary outcomes for infants and children; improved maternal health; and improved performance at school for children, among others. In addition to health benefits, WIC participants showed significant savings in health care costs when compared to nonparticipants.[30]

College Student Eligibility and Access to SNAP

There is a great deal of misinformation about college student eligibility for SNAP. Federal law limits the availability of SNAP benefits for college students attending more than half time unless they are working, are caring for children, or qualify for another exemption listed in the statute. This limitation, referred to as the SNAP student rule, is often referenced without referring to the long list of exemptions, which has led many students and practitioners to erroneously believe that all students attending college are ineligible.

Many low-income students qualify for exceptions, assuming they meet the SNAP income and asset criteria and one of the following criteria:

- working for pay at least 20 hours per week;[31]
- receiving, or having been awarded and anticipate receiving, any amount of federal or state work-study;
- caring for a child under age 6;
- caring for a child age 6–11 as a single parent while enrolled full-time or unable to obtain childcare;
- receiving TANF benefits;[32]
- unable to work because of a disability;[33]
- under the age of 18 or older than 50; or
- attending college as part of a Workforce Innovation and Opportunity Act (WIOA), Trade Adjustment Assistance (TAA), SNAP Employment and Training (SNAP E&T), or other state or locally funded training program, or equivalent.[34]

The 2014 Farm Bill limits state flexibility on the types of SNAP E&T programs under which a SNAP recipient may qualify for an exception. Specifically, it says that such a program must be part of a program of career and technical education (as defined under the Carl A. Perkins Career and Technical Education Act or Perkins Act) that may be completed in not more than four years.[35] Although new student rule regulations reflecting this 2014 change had not been published by December 2018, the intent of the law is to limit these programs to those that are employment focused.

Federal law gives the state SNAP agency the authority to decide what to count as equivalent to a training program. Many programs in community colleges could reasonably count as a state or local program for the purpose of employment and training. Massachusetts, Oregon, and Pennsylvania use the Perkins Act definition as a qualifier, so SNAP offices are not required to individually assess programs. The law also allows exceptions for SNAP E&T students enrolled in remedial courses, adult basic education, literacy, or English as a second language. The authors are not aware of any state that currently allows non-career-oriented enrollment in an institution of higher education, or postbaccalaureate education, to count as a SNAP E&T activity or equivalent.[36]

SNAP also imposes time limits for individuals who are considered Able-Bodied Adults Without Dependents (ABAWDs). These time limits apply to SNAP recipients ages 18–49 who do not live in households with children, are not pregnant, and do not have a mental or physical disability that would prevent them from working. This population captures some independent students without dependents who are not attending college more than half time. ABAWDs subject to the time limits may only access SNAP benefits for a total of three months in any 36-month period unless they are employed or are participating in a qualified work or training program (can include postsecondary) for at least 20 hours a week, or are participating in workfare for the required number of hours.[37] Unpaid or volunteer work also counts for the purpose of meeting the qualified work or training activity related to the ABAWD time limit, even though unpaid work does not qualify for an exemption to the student rule.[38] Students enrolled at least half time are exempt from the SNAP ABAWD time limit. However, students attending less than half time may be subject to the time limit.[39]

Implications for Student Financial Aid

Student aid programs included in Title IV of the federal Higher Education Act (HEA) use the Federal Methodology in determining eligibility for student financial aid and award levels. Pursuant to federal law, SNAP and WIC cannot be counted as income for the purposes of calculating students' Expected Family Contribution (EFC), which in turn determines the amount of federal financial aid for which students are eligible. Federal financial aid is largely not treated as income in determining eligibility for public benefit programs or benefit levels. Title IV of the HEA states that all federal student financial aid should not be taken into account in determining need or eligibility of any person for any benefits or assistance under any federal, state, or local program financed in whole or in part with federal funds.[40] Therefore, receipt of federal financial aid should not decrease the level of public benefits a low-income individual receives. While federal grant aid, including Pell Grants and Federal Supplemental Educational Opportunity Grants, applied to tuition and fees (or direct educational expenses) are never considered income, SNAP rules count as income any assistance that goes toward living expenses (or what is sometimes called indirect educational expenses). This can include food, lodging, books and supplies, and transportation.

Federal law draws a distinction between financial aid used for direct educational expenses—like tuition—and financial aid used for room and board. The regulations specify that federal financial aid for living expenses is countable as "income."[41] Financial aid, including student loans and federal and state work-study earnings, is not counted as income as long as it is used to pay for educational expenses, including tuition, books, and fees. Since TANF income is typically counted in determining eligibility and benefit levels under SNAP, states can count TANF-funded work-study earnings in the SNAP eligibility calculation, though this is an option that many states have not adopted.

Federal and State Policy Recommendations: Making Policy Changes

The federal government provides more than $122 billion a year in federal financial aid programs, but if students are unable to complete their degrees because of lack of basic needs, such as food, it puts the investment and the potential returns at risk. One cannot address the issue of college completion without addressing the issue of food insecurity. Different policy options exist to boost household income and to close the growing unmet need for all students—including increasing financial aid and the purchasing power of programs such as Pell Grants to keep pace with the true cost of college. But in the remaining parts of this chapter, the focus will be on how to improve students' access and use of SNAP and what potential federal and state changes to SNAP could meaningfully and effectively reduce food insecurity among students.

SNAP is the largest federal assistance program to combat food insecurity, funded at $68 billion annually, which is 25 times the total budget of the nation's largest charitable anti-hunger organization. Currently, SNAP helps 39 million Americans put food on the table every day. Studies show that SNAP receipt is an effective intervention to ameliorate hunger. It reduces food insecurity among recipients by as much as 30 percent and is even more effective among children and those with very low food insecurity.[42] SNAP allows low-income households to spend less of their very limited budgets on food, freeing resources that could go toward other basic needs. For students, the additional resources could be redirected toward education-related expenses.

Yet the 2018 GAO report found that among potentially SNAP-eligible, low-income students with at least one additional risk factor for food insecurity, an estimated 57 percent did not report participating in SNAP in 2016.[43] Low participation stems partly from federal program eligibility restrictions, but also from a lack of clarity regarding program eligibility rules at the state, county, and institution levels, where the administration of benefits—outreach, application, certification, and recertification—is done.

To understand existing SNAP restrictions for students and how to increase access and usage among today's students, one must first move beyond outdated ideas of who students really are. The typical student is no longer someone who enrolls in college immediately after high school, attends full-time, and can depend on their family for financial support. Indeed, such traditional students now make up just one-third of the college population.[44] Today's college students are increasingly low-income, working adults balancing work, family, and school. These students are also more likely to be first-generation attenders, immigrants, and students of color.[45] Nearly 50 percent of all students are living on their own and not financially dependent on their parents. A quarter of them have children. More than a third of low-income and first-generation college students and 37 percent of African American students, 33 percent of Native American students, and 25 percent of Latinx students are parents as well.[46] Most students work, either part-time or full-time, while enrolled in school in order to cover basic family needs such as housing, transportation, childcare, and food.

In the long run, many SNAP advocates and those supporting increased financial assistance for low-income college students would like to see the SNAP student rule lifted so that the program can serve and support today's college students using the same rules as for other program applicants and recipients. Given the political difficulty of achieving such a federal law change at this time, advocates hope that states will continue to implement the rule with the full consideration of its exemptions so as to maximize the existing flexibility and to ensure that low-income students who would benefit from SNAP and are eligible can more easily be served.

It bears emphasizing again that there is a misconception that the current SNAP student rule means that college students do not qualify for benefits. That is simply inaccurate—but clarifying the current rule and eligibility alone, while necessary and important, will not solve the problem of low enrollment in SNAP. Based on research and evaluation of other underenrolled populations—the elderly and the working poor—increased outreach and information did not meaningfully increase participation.[47] The more effective way is to simplify the application process for all applicants. However, it should be noted that having application assisters on campuses can serve the dual purpose of assisting with an application and identifying systemic and policy changes necessary to simplify the process for all student applicants, even those who do not benefit from having a campus-based application assister.

Federal Policy Recommendations

Protecting access and benefits for all eligible households also positively impacts those households with college students. The federal government should do the following:

- Increase the SNAP benefit. The average benefit provided by SNAP equates to roughly $1.40 per person per meal.
- Preserve current program flexibility and reject more restrictive measures such as onerous work requirements and time limits.
- Ensure that the WIC program has sufficient funding to meet all of the demand for benefits.

Over the past couple of years, members of Congress have grown more interested in addressing the deficiencies of the existing SNAP student rules, out of concern that it is barring access to those who could benefit most. Rep. Danny Davis (D-IL) sought to increase eligibility for foster and homeless youth through the Fostering Success in Higher Education Act, which he introduced in 2017. Rep. Al Lawson (D-FL) introduced the College Student Hunger Act in 2017. It proposed expanding the student eligibility rules to include more low-income students and those who have been determined to be independent, based on specified criteria included in the HEA. Neither bill was folded into the 2018 Farm Bill, but they did spur additional discussion about the inadequacy of the existing law in aiding the neediest students.

State Options: SNAP Student Rule Provisions, Maximizing State Flexibility

Many of the state policy recommendations for changes to SNAP entail encouraging states to maximize the flexibility already provided by the federal government in the existing statute:

- State SNAP agencies can develop guidance and training for state and college officials and staff on student eligibility rules, conduct outreach to local colleges and universities, partner with community partners to host office hours, screen students for eligibility, and host enrollment clinics on college campuses or areas with large populations of students.

- Most states have either raised or eliminated the asset limits to receive SNAP benefits. These asset tests are a huge administrative burden for state agencies and often penalize SNAP recipients for things like owning a reliable car worth more than $4,650 or having more than $2,250 in savings. Such low limits discourage and penalize long-term savings and economic mobility. While eliminating asset limits affects more than just students, rules such as vehicle asset limits can have a big impact on students who need their vehicle to get to and from school. Over 30 states exempt the entire value of the vehicle.[48]

- States have more flexibility than has generally been recognized to deem career-oriented postsecondary programs as equivalent to SNAP E&T programs and therefore allowable under the student exclusions. A promising model exists in Massachusetts, Oregon, and Pennsylvania, where the SNAP agency has determined that all community college programs that qualify for funding under the Perkins Act can be counted as education designed to improve employability. California has implemented a process by which programs can apply to be considered as an allowable exemption program, and it has approved programs for first-generation students, former foster care students, timed-out TANF recipients, and others. Such a practice promotes employment-focused education while removing a barrier to low-income students receiving SNAP. It simplifies low-income student eligibility for SNAP benefits significantly, without putting SNAP caseworkers in the position of having to make individual assessments of educational programs. This is a highly promising practice for replication.

- In order to improve student access to SNAP, simplify paperwork, and reduce churning on and off the rolls owing to work schedule variation, states should take the option of averaging hours of work across a month in determining whether a working student qualifies for an exemption from the student exclusion from SNAP.[49] This is particularly important given that many students have jobs with schedules that vary in hours by week. This is a clear best practice, as it both expands access and simplifies program administration.

- States should, to the extent possible, exclude state-funded work-study as income for SNAP. When it is counted, states should make sure to apply all appropriate exclusions. For instance, since this is a form of earned income, some states exclude 20 percent of earnings to cover work-related expenses.
- States should use their discretion to exclude all financial aid—federal, state, and institutional—as income from means-tested benefits where states have the discretion to define what is counted as income. It is not clear that all states understand their options to exclude state-funded work-study, either by blending it with federal work-study funds or by using the option to align SNAP income definitions to TANF.
- States should broaden the use of SNAP EBT for on-campus retail, online retail, and on-campus restaurants/prepared meals.
  - Only a handful of states participate in an RMP, which allows homeless, elderly, and disabled individuals to use their SNAP EBT card at participating restaurants. Recent research shows that roughly 13 percent of college students are homeless. Allowing these students to use their SNAP benefits for prepared foods would address their food insecurity.
  - Only a few college campuses accept EBT at their on-campus grocery stores and food retailers. This is partially due to the complexity of meeting the federal SNAP retailer rules. The federal government should provide technical assistance to colleges so more on-campus retailers can qualify for EBT.

- States can encourage institutions to inform all students who are eligible for or receiving federal or state work-study funds of their potential eligibility for SNAP.

Other Recommendations

States have other policy options beyond reforms to SNAP that they can pursue to help address student food insecurity and well-being:

- Postsecondary students should be provided with a basic meal guarantee. As part of a financial aid package, all colleges and universities should provide an allotment for 10 meals per week.
- Expanding SNAP access is one step toward overcoming the financial instability of low-income students. The federal and state governments also need to ensure broader access to subsidized childcare, Medicaid, and other financial supports. More money should be allocated for subsidized childcare, and policy barriers preventing low-income students from accessing these subsidies should be removed. In addition, those states that have not expanded Medicaid should do so, to ensure that more low-income students qualify for low- to no-cost health insurance.

Policy Change in California

Real change requires the right policies and the right politics. There are myriad possible paths toward improving SNAP access for eligible students. This is the story and the lessons learned from recent SNAP policy changes in California.

1. *Identifying "champions."*—It is critical to first identify leaders who understand the need for a policy response, can mobilize their constituencies, and are willing to share and leverage relationships, resources, and expertise. In California, the following diverse group of leaders is notable:

   - Samuel Chu, MAZON: A Jewish Response to Hunger, a political organizer who crafted and led numerous legislative and administrative campaigns around access to federal food benefits in more than 15 states.

- Jessica Bartholow, Western Center on Law and Poverty, with three decades of experience as the leading advocate for SNAP and public benefits access in California.
- State assemblywoman Dr. Shirley Weber, a former college professor turned legislator who authored a series of legislative proposals.
- Dr. Rashida Crutchfield, California State University (CSU) professor, who was principal investigator for the first CSU Chancellor's Office study on food and housing security and advocated for actions from within the university system.
- Ruben Canedo, Educational Opportunity Program and Food Security Committee at the University of California (UC), Berkeley, and a member of the UC Global Food Initiative Food Access and Security Subcommittee mobilized across campuses.
- Students: leaders from the UC Student Association, the CSU Student Association, and the Student Senate for California Community Colleges had a leading role in speaking out and testifying at the State Capitol.

2. *Create urgency and will for actions.*—Before the current growing body of research existed, advocates had to rely on anecdotal evidence and informal surveys to build the case that hunger is a growing problem on campuses. The emerging narratives and student voices, often well placed through media outlets, led to more formal and original system-wide research and surveys—quantifying the growing unmet needs and food and housing insecurity. Research studies from the UC and CSU systems that examined food insecurity among students helped build the case for policy change.[50] Together they created a fertile ground of political will and public urgency for legislative and administrative actions.

3. *Building power and a coalition through incremental "wins."*—The causes of food insecurity are complex, as are the solutions. No single "silver bullet" solution exists. At times the most strategic actions might have to be enacted by the state legislature, or changes implemented within the state's SNAP agency; other times, formal waivers must be sought by states from the USDA, or additional training of caseworkers must be conducted at county-level offices. Each incremental step provides an opportunity to recruit and train a different group of partners and allies, in ways that are aligned with their own unique political and economic interests and values. In California, actions were taken with key relation-

ships in mind and started where progress was possible even when it was limited:

- One of the earliest legislative proposals, Assembly Bill 1930 in 2014, created a work group within the California Department of Social Services, the department responsible for SNAP at the state level, to identify which "state or local job training programs" would exempt a college student from the student work rule. It was specific, targeted, and winnable.
- Another important step was correcting a widespread administrative oversight. While federal rules clearly exempt students from the SNAP student rule if they receive TANF-funded benefits, a majority of students receiving the TANF-funded benefits were not being ruled exempt. As a county-administered SNAP state, this required changes and retraining at the County Human Services agency level.
- More recent legislation created greater access to food on campuses for SNAP recipients who are disabled or homeless by increasing the likelihood that they can purchase a meal at a qualified food vendor on campus, beginning with the CSU campuses.

4. *Propagate best practices across states.*—States have the latitude to test and share ideas and best practices with each other. Though local reforms and state flexibility are vulnerable to shifts in federal policies, there has been successful replication of California's legislative and administrative actions in an increasing number of states. Similar SNAP-specific legislation has been passed in Illinois, and administrative reforms have been completed in Pennsylvania and Washington.

Conclusion

College is a key pathway to economic well-being. While college more accessible to students of color and first-generation and l income students than it was in the past, affordability can d even the strongest student aspirations. Many of these student overcome multiple barriers to arrive at college, only to have basic needs, such as food and nutrition, threaten their succ pantries can help address short-term hunger, but federal changes to SNAP and the WIC program will be necess that more low-income students have access to the federal supports necessary to thrive academically and complete college.

Acknowledgments

The authors would like to recognize Jessica Bartholow of the Western Center on Law and Poverty, who served as a reviewer of this chapter.

Notes

1. Anthony P. Carnevale, Stephen J. Rose, and Ban Cheah, *The College Payoff: Education, Occupations, Lifetime Earnings* (Washington, DC: Georgetown Center on Education and the Workforce, 2014), https://cew .georgetown.edu/cew-reports/the-college-payoff/.

2. Carnevale et al., *College Payoff*.

3. Anthony P. Carnevale, Nicole Smith, and Jeff Strohl, *Recovery: Job Growth and Education Requirements through 2020* (Washington, DC: Georgetown Center on Education and the Workforce, June 2013), https://cew.georgetown .edu/wp-content/uploads/2014/11/Recovery2020.FR_.Web_.pdf.

4. Anthony P. Carnevale, Tamara Jayasundera, and Artem Gulish, *America's Divided Recovery: College Haves and Have Nots* (Washington, DC: Georgetown Center on Education and the Workforce, 2016), https://cew .georgetown.edu/wp-content/uploads/Americas-Divided-Recovery-web .pdf.

5. Robert M. Kaplan, Michael L. Spittel, and Daryn H. David, eds., *Population Health: Behavioral and Social Science Insights* (Rockville, MD: Agency for Healthcare Research and Quality and Office of Behavioral and Social Sciences Research, National Institutes of Health, 2015); Jennifer Ma, Matea Pender, and Meredith Welch, *Education Pays 2016: The Benefits of Higher Education for Individuals and Society* (Washington, DC: College Board, 2015), https://trends.collegeboard.org/education-pays; Emily B. Zimmerman, Steven H. Woolf, and Amber Haley, "Understanding the Relationship between Education and Health: A Review of the Evidence and an Examination of Community Perspectives," in *Population Health: Behavioral and Social Science Insights*, ed. Robert M. Kaplan, Michael L. Spittel, and Daryn H. David (Rockville, MD: Agency for Healthcare Research and Quality and Office of Behavioral and Social Sciences Research, National Institutes of Health, July 2015), https://nam.edu/wp -content/uploads/2015/06/BPH-UnderstandingTheRelationship1.pdf.

6. William R. Emmons and Lowell R. Ricketts, *College Inadvertently Increases Racial and Ethnic Disparity in Income and Wealth* (St. Louis: Federal Reserve Bank of St. Louis, 2017), https://www.stlouisfed.org/publications /in-the-balance/2017/college-inadvertently-increases-racial-and-ethnic -disparity-in-income-and-wealth.

7. Kati Haycock, "Higher Ed's Pivotal Role in Breaking the Cycle of Poverty," *Education Trust*, May 28, 2015, https://edtrust.org/the-equity-line/higher-eds-pivotal-role-in-breaking-the-cycle-of-poverty/.

8. Doug Shapiro et al., *Completing College: A National View of Student Attainment Rates—Fall 2010 Cohort* (Herndon, VA: National Student Clearinghouse Research Center, 2016), https://nscresearchcenter.org/signaturereport12/.

9. Mamie Lynch, Jennifer Engle, and Jose Luiz Cruz, "Lifting the Fog on Inequitable Financial Aid Policies," *Education Trust*, Nov. 14, 2011, https://edtrust.org/resource/lifting-the-fog-on-inequitable-financial-aid-policies/; Patrick Reimherr et al., *Reforming Student Aid: How to Simplify Tax Aid and Use Performance Metrics to Improve College Choices and Completion* (Washington, DC: Center for Law and Social Policy, 2013), http://www.clasp.org/documents/Final-RADD-WhitePaper-Feb-2013.pdf.

10. US Government Accountability Office, *Food Insecurity: Better Information Could Help Eligible College Students Access Federal Food Assistance Benefits* (Washington, DC: US Government Accountability Office, Published Dec. 2018 and Publicly Released Jan. 2019), https://www.gao.gov/products/GAO-19-95.

11. Sandy Baum et al., *Trends in Student Aid 2017* (Washington, DC: College Board, 2017), https://trends.collegeboard.org/sites/default/files/2017-trends-student-aid_0.pdf; David Radwin et al., *2015–16 National Postsecondary Student Aid Study* (Washington, DC: Center for Law and Social Policy, 2018), https://nces.ed.gov/surveys/npsas/; "Poverty Guidelines," US Department of Health and Human Services, https://aspe.hhs.gov/poverty-guidelines.

12. Lauren Walizer, *When Financial Aid Falls Short: New Data Reveal Students Face Thousands in Unmet Need* (Washington, DC: Center for Law and Social Policy, Dec. 2018), https://www.clasp.org/sites/default/files/publications/2018/12/2018whenfinancialaidfallsshort.pdf.

13. US Government Accountability Office, *Food Insecurity*.

14. Sara Goldrick-Rab et al., *Still Hungry and Homeless in College* (Madison: University of Wisconsin HOPE Lab, Apr. 2018), https://hope4college.com/wp-content/uploads/2018/09/Wisconsin-HOPE-Lab-Still-Hungry-and-Homeless.pdf.

15. Goldrick-Rab et al., *Still Hungry and Homeless in College*.

16. Anthony P. Carnevale and Nicole Smith, *Balancing Work and Learning: Implications for Low-Income Students* (Washington, DC: Georgetown University Center on Education and the Workforce, 2018), https://cew.georgetown.edu/cew-reports/learnandearn/.

17. Rashida Crutchfield and Jennifer Maguire, *Study of Student Basic Needs* (Long Beach: California State University, Office of the Chancellor, Jan. 2018), https://www2.calstate.edu/impact-of-the-csu/student-success/basic-needs-initiative/Documents/BasicNeedsStudy_phaseII_withAccessibilityComments.pdf; Suzanna M. Martinez et al., "Food Insecurity in California's Public University System: What Are the Risk

Factors?," *Journal of Hunger and Environmental Nutrition* 13, no. 1 (2018): 1–18.

18. Derek Price et al., *Final Evaluation Report: Public Benefits and Community Colleges: Lessons from the Benefits Access for College Completion Evaluation* (Philadelphia, PA: Equal Measure, 2014), http://www.equalmeasure.org/wp-content/uploads/2014/12/BACC-Final-Report-FINAL-111914.pdf.

19. US Department of Agriculture, *Broad-Based Categorical Eligibility* (Washington, DC: US Department of Agriculture, Food and Nutrition Service, Oct. 2018), https://fns-prod.azureedge.net/sites/default/files/snap/BBCE.pdf.

20. "SNAP Eligibility," US Department of Agriculture, Food and Nutrition Service, https://www.fns.usda.gov/snap/eligibility#What%20deductions%20are%20allowed%20in%20SNAP.

21. US Department of Agriculture, *Supplemental Nutrition Assistance Program Caseload and Benefit Level Data* (Washington, DC: US Department of Agriculture, Food and Nutrition Service, Dec. 8, 2018), https://fns-prod.azureedge.net/sites/default/files/pd/34SNAPmonthly.pdf.

22. "Our Work," Feeding America, https://www.feedingamerica.org/our-work.

23. "Policy Basics: The Supplemental Nutrition Assistance Program (SNAP)," Center on Budget and Policy Priorities, https://www.cbpp.org/research/policy-basics-the-supplemental-nutrition-assistance-program-snap.

24. At the time of writing, Arizona, California, and Rhode Island administer RMPs.

25. 185 percent of the federal poverty guidelines was $22,459 for a family of one and $38,443 for a family of three, with slightly higher amounts for residents of Alaska and Hawaii. "7 CFR § 246.7—Certification of Participants," Cornell Law School Legal Information Institute, https://www.law.cornell.edu/cfr/text/7/246.7.

26. "Policy Basics: Special Supplemental Nutrition Program for Women, Infants, and Children," Center on Budget and Policy Priorities, https://www.cbpp.org/research/food-assistance/policy-basics-special-supplemental-nutrition-program-for-women-infants-and.

27. Each state is required to deliver WIC benefits via EBT cards by 2020.

28. "WIC Frequently Asked Questions (FAQs)," US Department of Agriculture, Food and Nutrition Service, https://www.fns.usda.gov/wic/frequently-asked-questions-about-wic.

29. "Policy Basics: Special Supplemental Nutrition Program."

30. "Special Supplemental Nutrition Program for Women, Infants, and Children (WIC): About WIC—How WIC Helps," US Department of Agriculture, Food and Nutrition Service, https://www.fns.usda.gov/wic/about-wic-how-wic-helps.

31. Many states have received a waiver allowing them to average hours of employment over a month. Schools may need to provide documentation of

hours of work to students employed as course assistants even if they are not paid on an hourly basis.

32. This may also apply to students who receive other TANF-funded benefits, such as childcare, diversion payments, etc.

33. Individuals who are unable to work because of disability are exempt from the student exclusion (and the three-month time limit). Meeting this exception does not require total and permanent disability at the level of Supplemental Security Income or Supplemental Security Disability Income eligibility.

34. "7 U.S.C. § 2015(e)," Cornell Law School Legal Information Institute, https://www.law.cornell.edu/uscode/text/7/2015; "7 CFR § 273.5—Students," Cornell Law School Legal Information Institute, https://www.law.cornell.edu/cfr/text/7/273.5; Elizabeth Lower-Basch and Helly Lee, *SNAP Policy Brief: College Student Eligibility* (Washington, DC: Center for Law and Social Policy, 2014), http://www.clasp.org/resources-and-publications/publication-1/SNAP_College-Student-Eligibility.pdf.

35. Note that this requirement is for the program, not the student. A program may only take four years for completion if pursued full-time but longer if pursued part-time.

36. "7 U.S.C. § 2015(e)—Eligibility Disqualifications," Cornell Law School Legal Information Institute.

37. "Workfare" is working in exchange for benefits.

38. US Department of Agriculture, *Supplemental Nutrition Assistance Program—ABAWD Time Limit Policy and Program Access. Memo to Regional Directors* (Washington, DC: US Department of Agriculture, Food and Nutrition Service, 2015), http://www.fns.usda.gov/sites/default/files/snap/ABAWD-Time-Limit-Policy-and-Program-Access-Memo-Nov2015.pdf.

39. Elizabeth Lower-Basch, *SNAP E&T 2014* (Washington, DC: Center for Law and Social Policy, 2014), http://www.clasp.org/resources-and-publications/publication-1/SNAP-ET-Overview.pdf.

40. "20 U.S.C. § 1087uu—Disregard of Student Aid in Other Federal Programs," Cornell Law School Legal Information Institute, https://www.law.cornell.edu/uscode/text/20/1087uu.

41. "7 CFR 273.9(c)—Income and Deductions," Cornell Law School Legal Information Institute, https://www.law.cornell.edu/cfr/text/7/273.9.

42. James Mabli et al., *Measuring the Effect of Supplemental Nutrition Assistance Program (SNAP) Participation on Food Security* (Washington, DC: Mathematica Policy Research for the US Department of Agriculture, Food and Nutrition Service, 2013), https://www.fns.usda.gov/measuring-effect-snap-participation-food-security-0; Caroline Ratcliffe, Signe-Mary McKernan, and Sisi Zhang, "How Much Does the Supplemental Nutrition Assistance Program Reduce Food Insecurity?," *American Journal of Agricultural Economics*, 93, no. 4 (July 2011): 1082–98, https://www.ncbi.nlm.nih.gov/pmc/articles/PMC4154696/.

43. US Government Accountability Office, *Food Insecurity*.

44. Lumina Foundation, *Who Is Today's Student?* (Indianapolis: Lumina Foundation, 2015), https://www.luminafoundation.org/files/resources /todays-student-summary.pdf.

45. Center for Law and Social Policy, *College Students Aren't Who You Think They Are* (Washington, DC: Center for Law and Social Policy, 2017), https://www.clasp.org/sites/default/files/publications/2017/08/2017June_ CollegeStudentsArentWhoYouThinkTheyAre.pdf; "Educational Profile," Community College Consortium for Immigrant Education, https://www .cccie.org/resources/fast-facts/educational-profile/; Emily Forest Cataldi, Christopher T. Bennett, and Kianglei Chen, *First-Generation Students: College Access, Persistence, and Postbachelor's Outcomes* (Washington, DC: US Department of Education, 2018), https://nces.ed.gov/pubs2018/2018421 .pdf.

46. Bethany Nelson, Megan Froehner, and Barbara Gault, *College Students with Children Are Common and Face Many Challenges in Completing Higher Education* (Washington, DC: Institute for Women's Policy Research, 2013), https://iwpr.org/wp-content/uploads/wpallimport/files/iwpr-export /publications/C404-College%20Students%20with%20Children%20 are%20Common%20and%20Face%20Challenges.pdf.

47. Jaqueline Kauff et al., *Reaching the Underserved Elderly and Working Poor in SNAP: Evaluation Findings from the Fiscal Year 2009 Pilots Final Report* (Washington, DC: Mathematica Policy Research, 2014), https://fns -prod.azureedge.net/sites/default/files/SNAPUnderseved-Elderly2009.pdf.

48. "Supplemental Nutrition Assistance Program (SNAP): Resources (Rules on Resource Limits)," US Department of Agriculture, https://www .snap-step1.usda.gov/fns/tool/tutorial/vehicle_states_chart/states_chart .html.

49. Because many students are likely to have part-time work with hours that vary, they may be unable to maintain 20 hours per week consistently to meet the eligibility requirement.

50. These studies included Rashida Crutchfield, *Serving Displaced and Food Insecure Students in the CSU* (Long Beach: California State University, Office of the Chancellor, Jan. 2016), https://presspage-production-content .s3.amazonaws.com/uploads/1487/cohomelessstudy.pdf?10000; Suzanna Martinez, Katie Maynard, and Lorrene Ritchie, *Student Food Access and Security Study from the University of California Global Food Initiative* (Oakland: University of California Office of the President, 2016), https:// www.ucop.edu/global-food-initiative/best-practices/food-access-security /student-food-access-and-security-study.pdf; University of California Global Food Initiative, *Global Food Initiative: Food and Housing Insecurity at the University of California* (Oakland: University of California Office of the President, 2017), https://www.ucop.edu/global-food-initiative/_files/food -housing-security.pdf.

Conclusion

KATHARINE M. BROTON AND CLARE L. CADY

Over the past decade, awareness of food insecurity and hunger on college campuses has increased dramatically. In many cases, increased awareness has been matched with action and intervention. Today, approximately 700 colleges and universities have campus pantries, and countless others have meal voucher programs, emergency grant aid initiatives, and one-stop shops that connect students to the public and private social safety net. Even more have joined networks like the College and University Food Bank Alliance and are committed to addressing food insecurity on their campuses. Practitioners, researchers, and policymakers come together to learn about the most promising approaches and share lessons learned in online platforms and at the annual #RealCollege Convening, a national conference hosted by the Hope Center for College, Community, and Justice.[1] In 2019, the federal government also acknowledged, for the first time, that food insecurity in higher education is a significant problem that must be addressed.[2]

The movement to end hunger on college campuses is growing, but there is much more work to do. Too many students attend college while struggling to get enough to eat, and others fail to enroll because of food insecurity. At the same time, research and evaluation efforts have not kept pace with the growing number of programmatic and policy efforts designed to support students and promote success. Research examining the causal impacts of intervention strategies is critical. If we are indeed going to address food insecurity as a student issue and try to end it, we need to know *what works* to ensure that students' needs are met so that they can reach their educational and life goals.

However, research on the efficacy of interventions is only one part of the research agenda necessary to truly address student hunger. We also need scholarship that provides us with a better understanding of the ways in which food insecurity manifests across students and institutional contexts and that investigates the connections among higher education, social, and economic policies and practices. Rather than view food insecurity as an individual attribute or characteristic, scholars, practitioners, and policymakers must investigate the systemic and intersectional nature of food insecurity in higher education in order to advance systemic solutions.

This book highlights some of the most promising strategies to end student hunger, drawing on insights from a diverse set of leaders in the field, but it simply cannot include all of the latest actions and interventions. Here we briefly describe three initiatives that have the potential to shape the movement to end student hunger in the coming years: the US Government Accountability Office (GAO) report on food insecurity among college students, the University of California Global Food Initiative, and two Hope Center experimental field studies examining food security interventions in higher education.

GAO Report on Food Insecurity among College Students

In January 2019, the federal government publicly recognized the substantial problem of food insecurity in higher education and stated that there is a role for federal and state policy in advancing solutions to end hunger on college campuses.[3] The report, done at

KATHARINE M. BROTON AND CLARE L. CADY

the request of Senators Debbie Stabenow, Patty Murray, Edward Markey, and Elizabeth Warren, reviewed extant research and practice and included the work of many scholars and practitioners featured in this book. The findings and recommendations echo much of what is said here: food insecurity is a serious issue undermining individual, state, and federal investments in higher education, and it must be addressed.[4]

Given the nature of the GAO, the report focused on the extent to which federal programs—and especially the Supplemental Nutrition Assistance Program (SNAP)—assist students experiencing food insecurity. The GAO's analysis identified 3.3 million students who were likely eligible to participate in SNAP in 2016 but found that just 43 percent, or 1.4 million, participated.[5] Thus, the report calls on the Food and Nutrition Service (FNS) to improve student eligibility information and share information on state SNAP agencies' approaches to help eligible students apply and participate in the program.[6] We agree that more needs to be done to connect the millions of eligible students to the existing social safety net, and SNAP in particular.

However, it is also clear that SNAP alone is not a sufficient response to the problem of food insecurity among students, and the report fails to interrogate the limitations of current SNAP policy. The report simply acknowledges that more than 1.3 million other students are at risk of food insecurity but are likely ineligible for SNAP assistance.[7] This estimate is almost certainly an undercount since the GAO analysis only focused on the 39 percent of domestic students with a household income at or below 130 percent of the federal poverty line.[8] While students from low-income families are more likely to experience food insecurity, the problem also affects those from moderate- and middle-income families struggling to afford the high price of college attendance, and the GAO report largely ignores this population. Many who anticipated this report hoped it would offer suggestions as to how policy change could make it easier for students to enroll in SNAP and other FNS programs, but it did not.

However, the very existence of this report validates the work of the field in that it provides federal recognition of the problem of food insecurity among students and its threat to student well-being and success. It is our hope that this report will be used as a step in the right direction in the areas of research, practice, and policy. Its call for additional research can serve to drive new scholarship, and its overview of practice can influence the spread of current interventions and inspire innovations in the work. It can also inform philanthropy to invest in both areas and bolster ongoing efforts to improve higher education and social policies.

University of California Global Food Initiative

Our colleagues in the University of California (UC) system are also taking a strong approach to addressing food insecurity among their students. In 2014, UC president Janet Napolitano, along with UC's 10 university chancellors, launched the UC Global Food Initiative—an intentional, systemic approach to "address one of the critical issues of our time: how to sustainably and nutritiously feed a world population expected to reach eight billion by 2025."[9] The initiative spans all 10 campuses, engaging in work on matters related to food production, access and security, sourcing, education and communication, and policy and public impact.[10] Since its inception, the initiative has produced more than a dozen reports and toolkits and actively engages in program development and policy change.[11]

Understanding and addressing basic needs insecurities across UC campuses has been a clear and active part of the UC Global Food Initiative. As the initiative started in 2014, a work group was formed to focus on this issue, and in 2015 they fielded the Student Food Access and Security Survey, one of the largest surveys of its kind at the time.[12] This survey indicated that 44 percent of undergraduate students and 26 percent of graduate students reported having experienced food insecurity.[13] The findings from the survey, released in 2016, helped spur the UC president to allocate $4 million to fund research, the creation of support services and educational programming, and engagement on all 10 campuses.[14]

As a part of this work, all UC campuses have either opened a campus pantry or worked to expand their existing pantry programs.[15] These pantries are not the end of the work, however. Many of the campuses have secured facilities to open basic needs hubs,[16] offering not only food for students but additional services such as support in applying for CalFresh (SNAP in California), food assistance programs, and education on healthy cooking and eating.[17] These food security offerings are complimented by other supports and services such as housing, creating a holistic approach to students' basic needs.[18] Some hubs also engage in awareness and advocacy campaigns, like the Hunger and Homelessness Awareness Week activities held on the UC Berkeley campus, as described in chapter 4 of this book. Many of these hubs have increased their offerings for students through partnerships with other programs mentioned in this book, including the College and University Food Bank Alliance and Swipe Out Hunger.[19] Much of the work being done in the UC system was reviewed and highlighted in the 2018 GAO report on student food insecurity.

The work occurring in the UC system is compelling not only because it is being done in an intentional and systemic manner but also because it operates inside of a larger context focused on food justice and security for all. This includes examining the issue of hunger as a scarcity of food and the factors that contribute to it, seeking to understand them and address them as root causes rather than focusing only on the symptoms. It also places the work within other movements tied to these root causes, including human and environmental justice. By structuring the work in this manner, the UC system may be developing ways to end hunger beyond their student populations, with impacts felt for those on and off campus.

Food Security Intervention Studies Conducted by the Hope Center

In 2017, Drs. Goldrick-Rab, Broton, and Hernandez launched the first experimental evaluations of basic needs interventions in higher education, including two promising approaches to addressing food insecurity and a third focused on alleviating housing insecurity. These field experiments are a bold step forward in moving the work on basic needs insecurity from the "problem" space to the "solution" space. All three programs were developed by community colleges and their partners based on their local needs, resources, and opportunities, illustrating the importance of cross-sector collaboration in the fight against hunger in higher education.[20]

Meal Vouchers at Bunker Hill Community College

Leaders at Bunker Hill Community College in Boston, Massachusetts, have long been aware that their students endure food insecurity, and a cross-functional Hunger Team coordinates a multipronged response, including a campus pantry, benefits access, emergency aid, and a meal voucher program. Building on the success and lessons learned from a pilot meal voucher program, the college worked with the Wisconsin HOPE Lab (now the Hope Center) to refine their efforts and implement the Meal Voucher Program (MVP). Rather than wait for students to come forward, the MVP identifies first-year students who are currently experiencing or at risk of food insecurity and provides them with a debit card to use in the campus cafeteria. Over the academic year, students receive $750 in additional food support. Because the need is so great, Bunker Hill is unable to offer this program to all students who need it. Therefore, among eligible students, 126 students were selected at random to participate in the program during the 2017–18 academic year. All students, including those not in the program, are eligible to participate in a wide range of academic and student support services provided by the college, including the other food supports listed above, discounts for public transportation, aid with waiving health insurance requirements, help completing the Free Application for Federal Student Aid (FAFSA), financial literacy workshops, and reminders regarding resume writing, transferring, job opportunities, and scholarships.

Currently, the evaluation team is tracking and analyzing the outcomes of both program participants and eligible students who were not selected to participate. Long considered the gold standard in education research, the experimental design enables the research team to estimate the causal impact of an on-campus food assistance program on community college students' academic success, including persistence and graduation. In addition to tracking academic outcomes using administrative data records, the team is also collecting information from student surveys and interviews to assess program implementation and examine impacts on general well-being, including improvements in sense of belonging or reductions in stress. The results will be of great interest to colleges across the nation that already provide meal voucher or "swipe" programs on their campuses, as well as to others interested in implementing this type of intervention. Furthermore, the evaluation will "shed some light on the potential impacts of expanding a free or subsidized meal program—like the one implemented in America's K–12 schools—to community colleges."[21]

Food Scholarships at Houston Community College

In partnership with the Houston Food Bank (HFB), Houston Community College (HCC) provides "food scholarships" to new and continuing students with limited financial resources. Again, because the need outpaces available resources, 1,000 students were randomly selected to participate in the program over the 2017–18 and 2018–19 academic years, while all students have access to additional academic and student support services. As part of HFB's Food For

Change program, participating students get groceries twice per month at food pantries set up in parking lots adjacent to HCC campuses. Distributed in a manner similar to farmers' markets, students have choices about the food they select, including fresh fruits and vegetables, frozen meat, milk, bread, grains, cereals, canned protein and peanut butter, eggs, and some canned goods.[22] The program emphasizes healthy eating based on dietary guidelines that recommend increasing fruit and vegetable intake while simultaneously reducing intake of saturated fats, salts, and sugars.[23] At each visit, students can select up to 30 pounds of fresh fruit and vegetables and 30 pounds of meat and dry goods; they also have access to cooking tips that correspond to available produce.

The research team is currently collecting administrative, survey, and interview data from both students in the program group and those who were eligible but were not selected for participation, in order to estimate the causal impact of the program on academic success and student well-being. An implementation study also tracks the amount and types of food that students select. Unlike many campus food pantry models, the food scholarship program proactively reaches out to students, helping them reduce grocery expenses while securing the nutritious food that they need. The results will be of considerable value to those interested in new approaches to collaborating with local food banks or looking to provide additional programming from their campus food pantry. Strategic partnerships like this one have the potential to offer benefits to both partners while producing support for students and their families.

Areas of Further Exploration

Addressing food insecurity and hunger on our college campuses requires a comprehensive and strategic plan. For some students, intermittent access to a campus food pantry may be enough to address their needs, while other students may require on-campus meal programs to alleviate short-term hunger. In some cases, the need goes way beyond what these programs can deliver, and access to additional resources, such as those in the public and private social safety net, is essential. When serving students who are currently struggling with food insecurity and hunger, there are a number of general approaches worth further exploration, including employing social workers to address students' needs, leveraging technology, and cultivating relationships with the business sector.

Social Workers

The strategy of hiring social workers for positions focused on addressing students' basic needs, as outlined in chapter 9, is not unique to Amarillo College (AC). Many campuses are employing social workers in integrated programs, as is the case at AC and in academic and student support services, such as in a counseling center or a dean's office. Social workers bring a different set of skills than those with higher education backgrounds in student affairs, for example. Social workers are trained to address human issues and consider both the whole person and their entire context when intervening to support a student. Social workers can also serve to blur the lines between campus and community, building extensive service networks that have the potential not only to connect students to additional off-campus resources but also to create pathways for members of the community to enroll in college as well. We do not yet know whether this approach is more impactful than other efforts to address student food insecurity, but we see it as an emerging strategy that needs further exploration.

Technology

In a digital age where so much of our work is automated and so much of our information comes to us through the internet, it is important to consider the role technology could have in addressing food insecurity among students. The most basic way technology is being utilized is through social media, both as a means to connect students to services and to promote interventions and programs addressing student food insecurity. The College and University Food Bank Alliance (chap. 2), for example, serves over 700 members with only a website and cell phones, indicating that technology can be leveraged to build capacity and to educate. Other organizations utilize an online platform created by Crew 2030 to engage with campus chapters and provide them with online trainings and tools to address food insecurity on their campuses (chaps. 4 and 5). More specialized approaches—like the Single Stop screener tool currently used in nine states (chap. 6)—are designed to connect students to particular resources. While these are great examples, there has yet to be a major push toward technological solutions addressing student food insecurity.

We doubt that technology will be able to solve this very human problem, but there is a role for it to play. For instance, we may be able to leverage technology to connect students to the social safety net. Is there a way to link students' FAFSA with SNAP applications, for example, building on lessons learned from the Internal Revenue Service Data Retrieval Tool? Given the range and diversity of students' food insecurity experiences and the need for multifaceted responses, we must consider ways to balance scale and scope with depth and intensity. Technological and other "low-touch" advancements in the field have the potential to complement the "high-touch" work of higher education professionals and social workers.

Partnerships with Business

Businesses are beginning to play a larger role in the movement to address food insecurity among students, and we should consider ways to effectively manage these relationships. Currently, many businesses provide food and monetary resources to programs and initiatives such as campus pantries and food swipe donation programs, as explained in chapter 5. These philanthropic efforts both are commendable and raise questions as to whether or not businesses can do more. The work at AC and Milwaukee Area Technical College (chaps. 3 and 9) provides examples of how businesses can support students and higher education institutions. When a utility company allows the college to pay a bill through their emergency aid program, or a mechanic will fix a car for a student today with payment coming from the college later, students' needs are met quickly, and the businesses only had to exhibit flexibility, trust, and patience. Employers of students can also serve to address student food insecurity by exhibiting these attributes. When employers commit to hiring students into jobs with work schedules that are flexible enough for students to attend classes, they make it possible for them to earn the money they need to afford all of the costs of college—including food. Employers who do this may also be able to retain their workers longer, and even promote them as they complete their studies. While none of these approaches are new, we see the potential to make a difference in the prevalence of food insecurity on a particular campus or within a particular community.

Root Problem of Food Insecurity among College Students

Part of any multifaceted approach to fight student hunger must also include provisions to prevent students from becoming food insecure in the first place. The roots of this problem lie in the changing economic structure of our society, in general, and higher education, in particular, coupled with reductions in the public social safety net. Today, adults with a college credential outperform their peers with a high school diploma on almost every measure of economic, social, and civic well-being—and the magnitude of these disparities has increased over time.[24] Simply put, it is increasingly difficult to lead a financially secure life without a college diploma, certificate, or degree. At the same time, the total price of college attendance has increased, while need-based financial aid and family incomes have stagnated.[25] As a result, students and their families must devote a substantial share of the total family income—often more than a quarter of it—to attend college.[26] Even though most students work and receive financial aid, a substantial number report that they cut back and skip meals or reduce the quality of their diet in order to try to make ends meet.[27]

Programs and policies that improve college affordability and reduce the *total* net price of college attendance (i.e., tuition and fees, room and board, books and supplies, and personal expenses) are critical to alleviating food insecurity and hunger on college campuses. Opportunities to implement free college programs, shore up declining state support for public higher education, and provide additional need-based financial aid should be understood as food insecurity interventions as well. Although these types of initiatives are not discussed at length in this volume, there is a relatively large and growing body of work dedicated to improving college affordability.[28]

Given the scope, depth, and complexity of the problem, however, higher education policies and programs are unlikely to end food insecurity and hunger on their own. Instead, efforts to increase family incomes and material resources for those with low and moderate incomes can also serve to promote food security. Again, this volume did not explicitly include broad efforts to raise wages, improve employment benefits, or strengthen the social safety net, but these types of initiatives are discussed elsewhere and can also improve food security in higher education.[29] Efforts to support the most vulnerable individuals in our society can spill over and directly assist those who are seeking a higher education. Similarly, on-campus efforts to support our most vulnerable students can improve the college experiences and outcomes of all students.

Recommendations for Practice

The problem of food insecurity and hunger in higher education can seem overwhelming, but everyone and every campus must start somewhere. Many institutions start with a campus food pantry—perhaps filled with donations—before establishing a partnership with a local food bank or adding other interventions described in this book. While we recommend that colleges and universities develop a multifaceted holistic approach to alleviating food insecurity on their campuses, the resources and relationships necessary to implement such an approach take time to develop and secure. Start by increasing awareness and implementing discrete actions, build from successes and lessons learned, and join in the movement.

Regardless of the exact food insecurity intervention or action, implementation matters. It is not just important that you *have* a campus food pantry or meal voucher program, for example. It is also important to consider *how* it is conceptualized, accessed, integrated, and maintained. This implementation must be student centered, using information from students on what they need and how they want it to be provided. Although food insecurity is not a particularly unique college experience, it still carries shame and stigma. Most people do not like to talk about it. Programs must be designed in ways that account for and address these and other barriers. We have found that students are often the best advisors in finding ways to make services more welcoming and inclusive. Additionally, the most promising practices appear to be those that are normalized and woven into the fabric of the college community, such as AC's Advocacy and Resource Center, described in chapter 9.

Furthermore, not all food is created equal. Humans have a complex relationship with food that exceeds the biological, including social, cultural, and religious practices. It is inappropriate for charitable initiatives to dump unhealthy, expired, and low-quality food on individuals in need. At the same time that we must honor individuals' autonomy and preferences, we must find ways to support a healthy and nutritious diet.[30] The Food Scholarship program in Houston is one example of how a food pantry model can encourage students to make healthy food choices.

Next, practitioners have a key role to play in strengthening the empirical foundation of food insecurity interventions in higher education. We strongly encourage you to track program data and use it in decision-making. At some institutions, institutional research offices may be able to support these efforts and help showcase relationships among program use, college investments, and student outcomes. In other cases, faculty and students may provide critical research support, as explained in chapter 8. Data and information have the potential to improve services on your campus, and when shared in professional networks, they can also directly shape the field.

Higher education practitioners are well positioned to alleviate food insecurity among college students, but they are unlikely to solve the problem on their own. It is simply too big and too complex. Therefore, we encourage practitioners to find ways to leverage external partnerships, including those with businesses, nonprofit organizations, government agencies, philanthropists, and civic organizations. Nearly every chapter in this book mentions a partnership or collaboration, highlighting the power of allies and networks in the movement.

Recommendations for Research

Scholarship has played and will likely continue to play an important role in addressing food insecurity in higher education. Research examining the prevalence of the problem and implications for student success has provided important motivation for action.[31] Results from multi-institution, system-wide, and statewide studies consistently report that substantial shares of students are food insecure and that these experiences are associated with poorer academic outcomes, but nationally representative estimates are not available owing to a lack of data.[32] The federal government must add comprehensive measures of basic needs insecurity to existing US Department of Education studies of college students, like the National

Postsecondary Student Aid Study, and find ways to account for individual college experiences among survey studies of the adult population.[33] Similarly, there is important work to do in terms of refining and clarifying survey measurement. Advancements in national data collection efforts are essential to furthering the study of basic needs insecurity in higher education and, ultimately, better serving students.

Although there is more work to do in understanding the problem of food insecurity in higher education, the takeaway is clear: food insecurity is a serious problem for a large number of college students, and we must find ways to address it. Researchers must turn from a sole focus on the "problem" space to an increased emphasis on the "solution" space. Currently, there is a tremendous opportunity for scholars to collaborate with practitioners and study what works for whom, under what conditions, and why. Ideally, these evaluations would track program participants or those affected by a new policy and a comparison group using a variety of methods, as described above, so that we can determine the efficacy of an intervention. We need research on *what works* and research that delves into the "black box" of intervention studies to understand which program components are best suited to serve which types of students or food insecurity experiences.

Beyond program and policy evaluation studies, basic scientific research has the potential to push the field forward in new and exciting ways. The issue of food insecurity in higher education lies at the intersections of scholarship on education, health, public policy, inequality, class mobility, and human rights. This provides countless opportunities for a diverse range of scholars to apply their theoretical understandings and methodological tools to the study of it. This work could be situated in a social or ecological framework that includes the contexts in which higher education food insecurity experiences are situated, including the groups or communities that are affected and those that could be engaged to promote food and basic needs security.[34]

Applied and basic research on food insecurity in higher education often benefits from cross-sector and multidisciplinary collaborations, given the complexity of the problem and need for multifaceted solutions. Translation and dissemination of research findings are also necessary to reach practitioners, as well as institutional and policy leaders and decision-makers. This type of work is difficult, is time-consuming, and can be expensive. Financial and in-kind support is critical to advancing the research agenda dedicated to understanding and alleviating food insecurity in higher education.

Recommendations for Policy

Changes in public policy are necessary to end student hunger and food insecurity. Currently, our social and education policies are not in alignment and fail to create a comprehensive system of support for students with basic needs insecurity who are pursuing a college credential.[35] In this volume, chapter 10 provides a series of detailed federal, state, and local policy recommendations designed to ensure that social and education policies work together to better support students. This includes short-term solutions intended to help make the current system work better and longer-term solutions that will require significant political will. For example, social policies— including FNS program rules—that utilize "college student" status as a meaningful category are outdated and fail to recognize the diversity and lived realities of today's college students. College student status is not an appropriate proxy for "well-off" or a convenient shortcut to exclude individuals from means-tested programs; this practice should be eliminated.

Overall, the problem of food insecurity and hunger among college students is rooted in the problem of college unaffordability. As the total price of college attendance has increased, need-based financial aid and family incomes have stagnated and the social safety net has frayed. Public policies must consider the full price of college attendance, including tuition and fees, room and board, educational supplies, and personal expenses, so that students are able to concentrate on their studies and learn. Improving college affordability, through any number of public policies, would go a long way toward alleviating food insecurity and hunger among students.

Despite increasing attention and awareness of food insecurity among college students, many people remain skeptical of the magnitude and severity of the problem. Stereotypical notions of the "starving college student" subsisting on a "ramen noodle diet" are often discussed as an appropriate and legitimate social rite of passage. Others disparage "students these days," questioning their financial choices and wondering why they cannot work their way through college like prior generations. In reality, most students work and receive financial aid, but the rising price of college, combined with stagnant wages and need-based financial aid, leaves even the most financially savvy students short of making ends meet. Food insecurity in higher education is not an individual characteristic but a systemic problem rooted in current education and social policies and practices.

Although there is public resistance to such efforts, policy changes that expand SNAP eligibility or extend the National School Lunch Program to higher education are likely cost-effective responses since undergraduates who receive public benefits are more likely to persist than observably similar peers who do not.[36] Increasing need-based financial aid can also improve graduate rates.[37] Given the substantial federal, state, local, and private investment in higher education and the moral imperative to support those seeking a college credential, we must take actions to alleviate food insecurity among students. Such steps have the potential to improve not only college attainment rates but also the health and well-being of our communities and nation.[38]

Notes

1. The Hope Center for College, Community, and Justice, founded by Dr. Sara Goldrick-Rab, is a nonprofit research center focused on rethinking and restructuring higher education and social policies, practices, and resources to create opportunities for all students to complete college degrees. The Hope Center seeks to improve the lives of #RealCollege students by redefining the status quo, drawing attention to those "nonacademic" issues that are often overlooked when evaluating higher education and other social institutions. Established in 2018, the Hope Center evolved from the Wisconsin HOPE Lab (2013–18), also founded by Dr. Goldrick-Rab with support from the Great Lakes Higher Education Guaranty Corporation. For more information, visit hope4college.com.

2. US Government Accountability Office, *Food Insecurity: Better Information Could Help Eligible College Students Access Federal Food Assistance Benefits* (Washington, DC: US Government Accountability Office, Published Dec. 2018 and Publicly Released Jan. 2019), https://www.gao.gov/products /GAO-19-95.

3. US Government Accountability Office, *Food Insecurity*.

4. US Government Accountability Office, *Food Insecurity*, 1.

5. US Government Accountability Office, *Food Insecurity*, 19.

6. US Government Accountability Office, *Food Insecurity*. Recommendations available at https://www.gao.gov/products/GAO-19-95#summary _recommend.

7. US Government Accountability Office, *Food Insecurity*, 19.

8. US Government Accountability Office, *Food Insecurity*, 15.

9. "Global Food Initiative: Overview," University of California Office of the President, https://www.ucop.edu/global-food-initiative/index.html.

10. "Global Food Initiative: Organization," University of California Office of the President, https://www.ucop.edu/global-food-initiative/organization /index.html.

11. "Global Food Initiative: Reports," University of California Office of the President, https://www.ucop.edu/global-food-initiative/best-practices /index.html.

12. University of California Global Food Initiative, *Global Food Initiative: Food and Housing Security at the University of California. Executive Summary* (Oakland: University of California Office of the President, 2017), 1.

13. Suzanna M. Martinez, Katie Maynard, and Lorene Ritchie, *Student Food Access and Food Security Study* (Oakland: University of California Office of the President, 2016).

14. University of California Global Food Initiative, *UC Efforts to Address Student Food and Housing Security* (Oakland: University of California Office of the President, n.d.).

15. University of California Global Food Initiative, *UC Efforts*, 1.

16. University of California Global Food Initiative, *UC Efforts*, 1.

17. "Food Support," UC Berkeley Basic Needs Hub, http://basicneeds .berkeley.edu/resources.

18. University of California Global Food Initiative, *UC Efforts*, 1.

19. University of California Global Food Initiative, *UC Efforts*, 1.

20. For more information, see Sara Goldrick-Rab, Katharine Broton, and Daphne Hernandez, *Addressing Basic Needs Security in Higher Education: An Introduction to Three Evaluations of Supports for Food and Housing at Community Colleges* (Madison: Wisconsin HOPE Lab, 2017), https://hope4college.com/wp-content/uploads/2018/09/Addressing-Basic-Needs-Security-in-Higher-Education.pdf.

21. Goldrick-Rab, Broton, and Hernandez, *Addressing Basic Needs Security*, 6.

22. Daphne Hernandez, "Food Scholarships Could Help More Students Finish College," *Conversation*, Mar. 5, 2018, https://theconversation.com/food-scholarships-could-help-more-students-finish-college-91615.

23. US Department of Health and Human Services and US Department of Agriculture, *2015-2020 Dietary Guidelines for Americans*, 8th ed. (Washington, DC: US Department of Health and Human Services and US Department of Agriculture, Dec. 2015), http://health.gov/dietaryguidelines/2015/guidelines/.

24. See, e.g., Clive R. Belfield and Thomas Bailey, "The Benefits of Attending Community College: A Review of the Evidence," *Community College Review* 39, no. 1 (2011): 46-68; Anthony P. Carnevale, Nicole Smith, and Jeff Strohl, *Help Wanted: Projections of Job and Education Requirements through 2018* (Washington, DC: Georgetown University Center on Education and the Workforce, 2010); Robert Haveman and Timothy Smeeding, "The Role of Higher Education in Social Mobility," *Future of Children* 16, no. 2 (2006): 125-50; Michael Hout, "Social and Economic Returns to College Education in the United States," *Annual Review of Sociology* 38, no. 1 (2012): 379-400; Philip Oreopoulos and Uros Petronijevic, "Making College Worth It: A Review of the Returns to Higher Education," *Future of Children* 23, no. 1 (2013): 41-65; Pew Research Center, "The Rising Cost of *Not* Going to College," Feb. 11, 2014, http://www.pewsocialtrends.org/2014/02/11/the-rising-cost-of-not-going-to-college/.

25. Sara Goldrick-Rab, *Paying the Price: College Costs, Financial Aid, and the Betrayal of the American Dream* (Chicago: University of Chicago Press, 2016).

26. Robert Kelchen, "Trends in Net Prices by Family Income," *Kelchen on Education* (blog), June 6, 2018, https://robertkelchen.com/kelchen-on-education/.

27. See chap. 1 for more information.

28. See, e.g., Goldrick-Rab, *Paying the Price*.

29. See, e.g., Matthew Desmond, *Evicted: Poverty and Profit in the American City* (New York: Crown, 2016); Kathryn Edin and H. Luke Shaefer, *$2.00 a Day: Living on Almost Nothing in America* (Boston: Houghton Mifflin Harcourt, 2016).

30. US Department of Health and Human Services and US Department of Agriculture, *2015-2020 Dietary Guidelines*.

31. See, e.g., work by the Hope Center for College, Community, and Justice at Temple University (formerly the Wisconsin HOPE Lab), University of California Global Food Initiative, and California State University Basic Needs Initiative.

32. US Government Accountability Office, *Food Insecurity*.

33. Lois Elfman reported that Kathryn Larin, director of the Education, Workforce, and Income Security Team of GAO, has stated that "there is a plan by the National Postsecondary Student Aid Study (NPSAS) to start including questions related to food insecurity." Lois Elfman, "GAO Report Tackles Issues of Food Insecurity among College Students," *Diverse Issues in Higher Education,* Jan. 9, 2019, https://diverseeducation.com/article/135731/.

34. See, e.g., Katharine M. Broton, Graham N. S. Miller, and Sara Goldrick-Rab, "College on the Margins: Higher Education Professionals' Perspectives on Campus Basic Needs Insecurity," *Teachers College Record* (forthcoming).

35. US Government Accountability Office, *Food Insecurity*.

36. For studies on public benefits and college success, see, e.g., Derek Price et al., *Public Benefits and Community Colleges: Lessons from the Benefits Access for College Completion Evaluation* (Philadelphia: OMG Center for Collaborative Learning, 2014), http://www.equalmeasure.org/wp-content/uploads/2014/12/BACC-Final-Report-FINAL-111914.pdf; Lindsay Daugherty, William R. Johnston, and Tiffany Tsai, *Connecting College Students to Alternative Sources of Support: The Single Stop Community College Initiative and Postsecondary Outcomes* (Santa Monica, CA: RAND Corporation, 2016), https://www.rand.org/pubs/research_reports/RR1740.html. For a policy proposal to expand the National School Lunch Program to higher education, see Sara Goldrick-Rab, Katharine Broton, and Emily Brunjes Colo, *Why the Time Is Right to Expand the National School Lunch Program to Higher Education* (Scholars Strategy Network, May 16, 2016), https://scholars.org/brief/why-time-right-expand-national-school-lunch-program-higher-education.

37. Benjamin L. Castleman and Bridget Terry Long, "Looking beyond Enrollment: The Causal Effect of Need-Based Grants on College Access, Persistence, and Graduation," *Journal of Labor Economics* 34, no. 4 (2016): 1023–73; Sara Goldrick-Rab et al., "Reducing Income Inequality in Educational Attainment: Experimental Evidence on the Impact of Financial Aid on College Completion," *American Journal of Sociology* 121, no. 6 (2016): 1762–817.

38. See, e.g., Belfield and Bailey, "The Benefits of Attending Community College"; Hout, "Social and Economic Returns"; and Oreopoulos and Petronijevic, "Making College Worth It."

Congressional Hunger Center, 107
Conley, Lisa, 69, 72
Conoley, Jane, 194
consultant approach, 36, 120-21
Cooperating Agencies Foster Youth
Educational Support, 129
corporate social responsibility, 136
Covenant House California, 193
Craig, Raven, 211-12
Crew2030 initiative, 98, 274
Crutchfield, Rashida, 168, 193-95, 205,
206, 208, 258. See also *Study of
Student Basic Needs* (Maguire and
Crutchfield)
cumulative advantage and disadvan-
tage theory, 197-98
customer relationship management
technology platform, 131
customer service, 229

Dance Marathon program, 105-6
data collection and analysis, 47-48,
49, 100, 131-33, 143, 150, 278
Davis, Danny, 254
Deferred Action for Childhood
Arrivals (DACA) students, 64, 66,
69-70
Delgado Community College, New
Orleans, 146
Desmond, Mathew, 58, 60, 63-64
"diploma mills," 76-77
disabled students, 246-47, 249, 256, 259
Dowell, David, 194

education, as positive externality, 76
elderly students, SNAP use, 246-47, 256
Electronic Benefit Transfer (EBT), 177,
183-84, 214, 215, 246, 256
emergency aid programs, 5, 14, 126,
143, 153-54, 265; Blue Love Foundation, 146; Dreamkeepers, 56, 64-67,
68, 71, 72, 77-79
Emerson National Hunger Fellows
Program, 107
employed students, 15, 16, 19-20,
25n16, 243, 281; SNAP eligibility,
249, 250, 252-53, 255-56
Enlight Foundation, 98-99, 100

enrollment, opportunity costs of, 49
environmental movement, 104
*Evicted: Poverty and Profit in an
American City* (Desmond), 60, 63-64
Expected Family Contributions, 250

faculty, 2-3, 71-74, 202, 278
Faculty and Students Together (FAST)
Fund, 8. *See also* American Federation of Teachers Local 212/MATC
FAST Fund
Farm Bill, 249, 254
farms and gardens, for food production, 155, 205-7
Federal Supplemental Educational
Opportunity Grants, 251
Feeding America, 105, 135-36, 246
feminine hygiene products, 234
financial aid, 15-17, 19, 78; 150 percent
rule, 55, 61, 64, 66, 75-77; inadequacy,
16, 17, 24n12, 139, 242, 243-44, 275-76,
281. *See also* Pell Grants
financial independence, 15-16, 24n12
first-generation college students, 18,
55, 198, 200-201, 226, 253, 255
food, nutritional content, 272, 277
Food and Nutrition Service, 267, 280
food banks, local, 39, 40-43, 44-45,
118, 147, 178, 183, 215, 233, 272
food insecurity, 1-10, 15-17, 18-19, 20;
adverse health effects, 7, 20-21, 200,
201; categories, 18; definition, 17, 243;
federal government's recognition of,
266-68; high-risk groups, 18-19,
26n22, 232, 236; rate, 17-19, 18-20,
21-22, 26n22, 119, 172, 200, 226, 236,
243; as systemic problem, 266, 281
food insecurity interventions: benefits
of, 14-15; context, 2; implementation, 277; multifaceted approach,
2-3, 14, 52-53, 277; pros and cons, 2;
replication, 5, 10n2; selection, 3-4
food pantries, 4-5, 8, 10n3, 14, 91-92,
246, 259-60; Amarillo College,
232-34, 237-38; California State
University, 175, 178-79, 182-83; data
collection function, 47-48, 49;
dedicated space for, 43-45, 50;

surveys (*continued*)

    participation, 48, 50–51; #RealCol-lege, 48, 231; Student Food Access and Security, 268–69. *See also* Hope Center for Community, College, and Justice; Wisconsin HOPE Lab

Swipe Out Hunger, 9, 115–37, 269; case studies, 123–27; challenges, 128–30; collaborative approach, 104–5; evaluation, 131–33; expansion, 120–23; founding, 116–19; funding, 127, 128–29, 133–34; legislators' participation in, 133–35; organizational model, 121, 122; pilot program, 128–129; strategies, 120–23; Swipe Drive, 116

Swipes for the Homeless, 117–18

tax credits, 157–58

technology, 97–100, 273–74

Temple Association of University Professionals, 74

Temple University, Hope Center for College, Community, and Justice, 22, 37–38, 48, 50–51, 265, 282n1

Temporary Assistance for Needy Families (TANF), 245, 247, 249, 251, 255, 259

textbooks, 69, 152, 153, 158, 162, 251

Tinoco, Carolyn, 20

transcripts, 80

transportation, 161, 226, 230–31, 232, 251

triage, 174–75

TRiO-funded programs, 152

tuition, 15, 64, 152, 242, 251

undocumented students, 149, 152–53

US Department of Agriculture, 18, 147, 150, 183–84, 243, 246, 248

US Department of Education, 21, 242, 278–79

U.S. News & World Reports, 129

US Student Association, 110

US Supreme Court, *Janus* decision, 74

University of Arkansas, 36

University of California, 21, 38, 86, 188, 243, 258, 268–69

University of California, Berkeley, 85, 94–95, 258

University of California, Davis, 92

University of California, Irvine, 133

University of California, Los Angeles, 116–19

University of California, Santa Barbara, 123–24

University of Massachusetts, 146

University of Pennsylvania, 110

University of Southern California, 119–20

University of Wisconsin, HOPE Lab, 19, 21, 22, 226, 231, 269. *See also* Hope Center for College, Community, and Justice

University of Wisconsin-Madison, 91, 92

University of Wisconsin-Milwaukee, 57

unmet need, 242, 251–52

USA for Africa, 89

validation theory, 198–99

Warren, Elizabeth, 266–67

Waukesha County Technical College, 68–69

Weber, Shirley, 214–16, 258

Weinstein, Michael, 141–42

Western Center on Law and Poverty, 258

White, Maggie, 187, 188, 203–4

White, Timothy P., 168–69, 172, 173–74, 199, 218

Winkelman, Eli, 89

Winston-Salem State University, 146

Wisconsin Covenant Scholars Grant, 55–56

Wisconsin Energy Assistance program, 65, 71

Wisconsin HOPE Lab, 19, 21, 22, 226, 231, 269. *See also* Hope Center for College, Community, and Justice

Wisconsin Technical College system, 55

women's centers, 109

wraparound services, 5, 9, 13, 142

Yale Law School, 101–2